From the Brink of the Drink

A PERSONAL STORY OF TRIBULATIONS AND
TRIUMPHS OF ALCOHOLISM

Karla Juvonen

BRIGHTON PUBLISHING LLC
435 N. HARRIS DRIVE
MESA, AZ 85203

FROM THE BRINK OF THE DRINK

A PERSONAL STORY OF TRIBULATIONS AND
TRIUMPHS OF ALCOHOLISM

KARLA JUVONEN

BRIGHTON PUBLISHING LLC
435 N. HARRIS DRIVE
MESA, AZ 85203

WWW.BRIGHTONPUBLISHING.COM

COPYRIGHT © 2019
ISBN 13: 978-1-62183-540-0
ISBN 10: 1-62183-540-5
PRINTED IN THE UNITED STATES OF AMERICA

First Edition

COVER DESIGN: TOM RODRIGUEZ

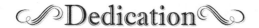Dedication

"This book is dedicated to the alcoholic still struggling."

Acknowledgments

This book, and my life as I now know it, would never have been possible if not for the support, love, and efforts put forth by so many people. I would like to thank my parents and my sister for loving me throughout this entire ordeal, even when I truly did not deserve it. Tami, Maureen, Jeanne, Patty, and Lauren–you are my rocks. Judy, my sponsor, thank you for always being there for me. I could not do this without you. I thank my ex-husband, Jim, for encouraging me to write this book, and for working with me to raise our beautiful kids in a healthy and peaceful partnership. Erik–I love you, I thank you, and I am so proud of you. Your support gets me through each and every day. To get this book out there, I am so grateful to Don McGuire at Brighton Publishing for taking a chance on an unknown writer, and to Chandler and Jimmy for pointing me in the right direction. To my beautiful children–Nick, Tate, Olivia, Evelyn, and Sawyer–I love you all. You are my reasons for continually trying to better myself and be the mother you deserve. Thank you to everyone at the Thursday night HCP recovery meeting, for support that is so constant and true. Most importantly, thank you God, for forgiveness, grace, and your constant presence.

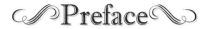Preface

THE END OF THE DRINKING

"**D**o you need help," asked Phil?

A slurred and mumbled response from an unrecognizable me followed with "yes, but I don't think I'm worth it. I think I'm a lost cause."

Phil, a guardian angel of sorts whom I spoke to only once, whose last name I don't believe I ever knew, quietly said "nobody is a lost cause."

Phil's 800 number had popped up on my computer screen. For some reason unknown to me still to this day, I called it instead of taking the mixture of pills in my hand that I was certain, based on foggy, drunken internet research, would kill me. Following a twelve-month period of time in which I had failed three detox's and two inpatient rehabilitation stays, had a messy divorce finalized and ended an affair of three years with my ex-husband's married boss. I also lost my job as a Physician Assistant, lost my medical license, lost the ability to see my children, was on the brink of losing my home and facing certain financial ruin. I had alienated nearly my entire family and friend network, began and ended a romantic affair with someone just as addicted as me which resulted in a pregnancy and abuse as well as a horrific and painful loss of a baby that was undoubtedly going to be born with fetal alcohol syndrome to two addicted parents—suicide seemed the only option. I was broken. Beyond repair. I did not feel "savable," nor did I feel worthy of being saved.

I could not stop drinking. I physically and psychologically simply could not stop, despite the fact that it had destroyed my life. I could not understand why. I should be able to put down the drink. I should be strong enough and have enough willpower to stop. I was educated and intelligent yet could not outsmart this. I had veered so far from the person I once was, that I could not look at myself in the mirror. If I happened a glance, it was full of self -loathing. My morals were nonexistent. I was a drunk, a liar, a manipulator, a failure as a mom, a failure as a human being. My priority list was short and included only vodka. I was disgusted with myself. How could I deserve any help? Is redemption even possible when one has gone so far off the grid?

Sobbing, I tried to relay my feelings of hopelessness to Phil. I was lying on the floor of my walk in closet with my 1.75 liter of vodka, my laptop, and my phone. In my 5900 square foot home, the closet was where I spent the majority of my time. People joke about "closet drinkers."

My alcoholism had made my life so small and I had become so isolated, that I was a literal closet drinker. I was horrified at what I had become, yet was clinging to the bottle because it was all I felt that I had left. Phil assured me that there was another way. He must have stayed on the phone with me for two hours, an attempt to solicit rehab business turned into a suicide intervention. At the end of the phone call, he had arranged a rehabilitation placement 2000 miles from home that would accept my insurance without any money down, as well as a plane ticket and a taxi to get me to the airport. It was a whirlwind. I stumbled about my home, throwing random things in my largest suitcase while continuing to drink. I called the only person who was still taking my calls although warily—Mom. She encouraged me as always. She let me know she would make sure the house and the cats and every other excuse I was using as a reason not to go, would be taken care of. "Just go, Karla," she said. She said she would do anything to help me get sober and stay that way. She pleaded with her voice filled with tears, anger and frustration. She told me I was worth it and that she would never give up on me. She asked me what I had to lose by going. Absolutely nothing, I had already lost it all.

So I went.

The poor cab driver did not know what he was in for. There it was, not even noon on a bright and sunny below zero Minnesota morning and he had been tasked with picking up this disheveled, emotional drunk woman.

Having run out of vodka, I instructed him to stop at a bar on the way to the airport. I lied and told him I hated flying and needed some liquid courage. In my stupor, I asked if I could buy him—my CAB DRIVER—a drink. He politely declined and decided, wisely, to wait in the cab for me. I pounded three double shots of vodka faster than the bartender could pour them. I paid with a credit card that I had no way of paying back. I did not care how it looked, I did not care that I couldn't afford it, I did not care that it was killing me. I needed it.

Upon arrival and check-in at the airport, I got through security without complication. I immediately found a bar and began ordering shots. I told people at the bar I was on my way to Florida for serious cardiovascular surgery and didn't know if I would make it, so I was celebrating in case it was my last time to drink. It was, of course, life or death—but I couldn't admit to anyone, least of all myself, that it was solely because of the alcohol.

Boarding time approached, and somehow I kept my wits about me enough to get to the gate. I tripped and fell on the jet way, to the horror of those around me. I was a yard sale. Coat here, bag there, purse way over there, contents of what remained of my sad life spilled all around my sprawled out drunken self. They still let me on the plane. And, they still let me immediately order and receive two of those tiny bottles of vodka while filling out an airline incident report. I continued to drink throughout that flight. There was a layover in Philadelphia, for which I was grateful because that meant invariably another bar. From my position on the bar stool, drinking vodka, I called my friend Lauren. I had met Lauren in my most recent inpatient rehabilitation stay, only a few weeks previously. She had remained sober. Clearly I had not. I slurred out to her what I was doing. She asked she recalls as the most stupid question she's ever asked in her life, "are you drinking." Of course! That's all I did. She kept on the line with me, asking when my connecting flight boarded, urging me to get to the gate, and that whatever I did I must not miss that flight. I thought I was in Atlanta. I was in Philadelphia. I thought I was cool and collected, I was anything but. I thought perhaps my situation really wasn't this bad and maybe I didn't really need this. She reminded me that I absolutely did. She told me that if she, who was also battling a type of breast cancer with only a 5% survival rate at ten years could stay sober, so could I. Ultimately, I made the connecting flight and continued to drink, even ordering another two of those tiny bottles to put in my purse for later. Arriving in Orlando, my final destination, I went immediately to the restroom before meeting my transport to the rehab facility. I drank those last two bottles—in a dirty toilet stall; all alone. That is where alcoholism had taken me. To the toilet, literally. That was the last time I ever drank.

✑Introduction✑

This is a story of self- discovery—an honest, fearless inventory of my past, learning to avoid my personal pitfalls and work on my character defects to become a better person. An attempt to not repeat the mistakes of my past; to learn to be happy in life. In my humble opinion, this is a much more important part of recovery than actually quitting the drink.

I don't know why I was given a second chance when so many others are not. It can only be the Grace of God and that, for some reason, I am still needed on this planet. I intend never to take my life for granted again.

Not for one minute could I have done this alone. It would have been impossible. Alcoholism and addiction isolated me. It lied to me, it told me I did not have a problem, or if I did, it really wasn't that bad. It told me I couldn't trust other people. It is a cunning, baffling disease, as stated in the Big Book of Alcoholics Anonymous. It was just as baffling to me as it was to those around me who loved me and could not understand why I kept doing this to myself. I couldn't understand either. At the end of my drinking, the very thing that was sustaining me on a daily basis was killing me slowly, painfully, and with an unimaginable amount of destruction in my wake. It tried to kill me emotionally, spiritually, and physically. For some reason, I fought back. And I am winning—one day at a time. I wrote this memoir in the hopes that someone out there struggling may find hope and determination in reading it.

I have been brutally honest in this book with exception of two specific situations which, if disclosed, would harm other people. Otherwise, honesty is the only way for me to do this—otherwise it would be a work of fiction, which this is most definitely not. My disclaimer however, is that during the last eighteen months of my drinking, things were obviously fuzzy and as I attempted to document events, my recollection may be slightly different than reality; different from the recollections of those who love me. Because, as you now know, I was a hopeless drunk. Or so I thought.

Much of what follows is part of the program of the 12 Steps. While I am not affiliated with any sect, denomination, AA, NA, state or national medical board, or monitoring agency, I do utilize and refer to literature from AA and NA including the 12 steps, and the Big Book of Alcoholics Anonymous, which from here on will be referred to as "the Big Book." If you are in a recovery program, or love someone who is, perhaps the Steps and little cliché sayings will be quite familiar. My story may seem much worse than yours leaving you feeling that you don't really have a problem. Or, your story may seem much worse than mine, making you feel like you can't relate. I have learned to try very hard not to compare my life or my story to anyone else's. My hope is that you can see this for what it is intended; a personal story of rise and fall and rise again within addiction. I am no better or worse than anyone else, in or out of the program. And neither are you. We are all human beings, with flaws and strengths. If at times I seem arrogant or self-deprecating, that's good—because I was both of those things; a dichotomy in my brain bouncing back and forth between ego and false pride, and self-hatred.

The good news is, I am no longer arrogant, I am confident when appropriate. I am no longer filled with ego or pride, though those are two character defects that I need to keep in check on a daily basis. I have pride in the real things in my life, without pride in stupid surface, fake things. My ego is fragile and easily bruised something I am now aware of and can manage. I do not hate myself anymore. And, I am only self-deprecating sometimes now. I have made so many bad choices and so many mistakes in my life, but have learned that bad deeds don't always equal a bad person. Sometimes, good people just do bad things. I wish I could change the past, but I can't. So, as the big book says, "we don't regret the past, nor wish to shut the door on it." I never want to forget where my alcoholism got me or repeat any of those chapters, but I no longer live in the guilt and shame of my past. I have learned from it, and continue to learn daily. Writing the majority of those instances down in the following pages is the epitome of vulnerability, and I am fully aware that I may be judged, hated, condemned, and criticized by many because of my past. And that's OK, I expect it. I did some really awful things and made one bad decision after another.

It may also be evident at points in this book that I was not a good mother and was endangering my children. That is true. I was a terrible mother during the worst of my addiction. Perhaps it may even appear that I didn't love my kids. Please don't make a mistake about that, because I loved and still love them more than life itself, so much so that I believed at the end that I would be doing the best thing for them if I simply killed myself. I am painfully honest about what kind of a mother I was when I was hopelessly addicted in the hopes that another parent can read my story and learn from it—and maybe stop their own disease progression.

I don't mean to come off preachy or "all-knowing" because I most certainly am not. And I don't believe that a 12 step program is the only way to get and stay sober. Some use a 12 step program, others utilize mediation assisted treatment (MAT). I know many people who have been able to control the use of their drug of choice with a harms reduction program. There is hypnosis, counseling, support groups, cognitive behavioral therapy, specific recovery programs, or a combination of many tools. Some are able to quit cold turkey. Others require detox, inpatient rehabilitation, or outpatient treatment. There are people who get and stay sober the first time they try, but the majority of us have several attempts under our belt. I know people who are sober from their drug of choice, but are still able to utilize prescribed medications, or even drugs or alcohol without destroying their lives or hurting other people. Some people believe that abstinence from all mood-altering substances is the only "real" recovery and that if someone is taking even a prescription sleep aid or antidepressant, they are not truly sober. Others are of the school of thought that whatever you need to do to stay off your drug of choice is recovery. Just as every addict and alcoholic is unique, so is their program of recovery. I am simply sharing my journey, and the tools that I utilize to stay away from drinking. I am not advocating that my program is the best or only way. It's just the program that works for me.

ᴄᴾChapter Oneᶜᴼ

The Beginning

I was born as the first child, the golden child, to my successful parents. Mom was a respected RN and my father, a successful crop farmer. A colicky baby for apparently my first ten months of life, my parents still decided to try again and my beautiful sister arrived three years later to complete our family. Success and appearances were important. Real or perceived, I felt that I must do well, be perfect, succeed, and definitely not rock the boat in any way. The early years that I am about to describe in NO WAY place any blame on anyone else regarding my eventual alcoholism. That is mine and mine alone, but the details are important in order to give a clear picture of who I am and how I got to where I got.

My father was stressed and quick to anger in those days, and I took it upon myself to try to ensure that he would have no reason to be angry at me. That if I just did well, he would be happy and not angry. My sense of self-importance was shockingly high at such a young age, and an ominous indicator of things to come. I felt that my parents expected perfection in all things, and felt that withdrawal of love was the punishment if I did not comply.

My successes were a direct reflection on them, and any failure (though I never failed in those days) would have been a reflection on them as well. This was never relayed to me by them, it was something I felt—a deep-rooted feeling of inadequacy. I became the peacemaker and people pleaser from as early as I can remember. A chameleon of sorts, my non-overt manipulation began early. Always saying what I thought people wanted to hear, rather than what I really felt. Changing my behavior and opinions based on who I happened to be with was my way, and I was good at it. It was a surefire recipe for losing myself at some point in life, though it was a slow burn for years until I realized it.

The days of glory for my successful family were short lived, however. During the 1980's, the farm crisis that swept through the Midwest laid claim to our farm. My dad and his brothers lost their beloved farm, and with it, I believe, their identity. They also lost their brotherly relationships, and two of them do not speak to this day. My mother stepped up even further work-wise to make ends meet financially. My dad buried himself in volunteer work within the community and eventually began driving a school bus and providing custodial services for the school. It was even more important to me to be "a good girl" and to please them. My sister and I divided up the house and yard work, had a lot of responsibilities and did what was expected of us. Me, with a false smile, gusto and a sickeningly positive attitude. Her, begrudgingly. See, she was a lot healthier as a kid than I was. She didn't buy in fully to the idea that pleasing everyone but yourself was the way to go. So, she bucked at times, and during those times I secretly was relieved it was her and not me in trouble, and relished the constant comparisons my parents made between the two of us. I was always better. That made me feel good, important, worthy, and determined to stay on that path. Straight A's followed, early success musically and in the theater, teacher's pet in many classrooms—being "the best" was my goal. Anything less would disappoint my parents, in my opinion, and they could not take any more disappointment or stress. Even in my diary, age nine, I wrote a passage "I am saving my money in case we get poor. We are having the oxen (auction, to a nine-year-old) tomorrow and everyone is sad. I need to be happy and not make problems." I put a great deal of pressure on myself to fit this role and these expectations, and did not understand until I finally became sober at age thirty-nine, that I really wasn't that important and that my behaviors, successes, and failures did not create someone else's happiness or misery. That was up to them, just as my own happiness or misery, is solely my own.

My parents drank, and still drink socially. We always had liquor in the house, but they would often go many days or weeks between episodes of drinking. Holiday celebrations intimately within our own home and those with extended family did not involve alcohol. It just wasn't a big deal to them. They enjoyed it on occasion, in moderation, and once in a while to excess. I was observant of these times. I noticed that adults who drank became funny and silly and relaxed in a way that I didn't usually see them. It was nice. I had a glorified idea of what alcohol could do for a person, and I began imagining myself being old enough to drink.

My sister and I were often alone at the house, with both parents out and about. I vividly recall cranking a vinyl record of "The Oak Ridge Boys," while pretending the dining room was a bar, and I was the waitress. I would bring out a tray with champagne glasses of ginger ale to serve to my "customer"—my sister. Then I would pretend that my job as a waitress was so stressful, and I would sneakily guzzle one or two of the glasses and begin to act relaxed and silly. I would also pretend that when my shift was over, I would go back to my "apartment"—my room, which I pretended to lock with a key, and relax with some more "champagne." My ideas of drinking were clearly not normal or healthy, from a very young age. I can think back now and see that I was already craving a way to escape from life, something to get me out of my own head; something to take the edge off, numb things, take away my anxiety and allow me to sleep. It seemed to work for the grown ups—maybe it would work for me, too.

It did.

Most alcoholics can say that they recall their first drink. I am no different. Inflicted with the chicken pox, and having them pop up in my mouth and throat as well as all over my skin, my parents made a regular strength grasshopper for me to try to relax and soothe. It worked. I remember that creamy, minty milkshake with the burning

4

aftertaste coating my mouth and throat, and warming me quickly from the inside out. It was almost magical. I slept well for the first time that I could remember. Sleep had been elusive for me since birth, according to my mother. Colicky at first, then just a poor sleeper, she would apparently put me down for the night or a nap, and come to check an hour or two or three later and I would be there— wide-awake. I was behaving, not making noise or a mess, but certainly wasn't sleeping.

So alcohol could help me with sleep—hallelujah! Now, if I could just figure out how to get more.

Never fear, I was smart and sneaky, still am. At twelve, I enjoyed a champagne fountain at a wedding with a cousin of mine. I quickly learned, however, that for me drinking was most delightful when I was alone—another red flag. I enjoyed the blissful numb solitude, and also enjoyed the fact that the risk of being caught decreased exponentially when I was not drinking with anyone else who could blow my cover or get me in trouble. I did not want drinking to screw up my success or my parents' view of me. I did not want to get in trouble at school or get in any trouble whatsoever. Best to do this one, for the most part, independently.

⟡Chapter Two⟡

THE TEENAGE YEARS

I t began late at night when everyone else was asleep in the house. I would creep to the liquor closet, which was in my father's office. It was big enough to walk into. I would pour enough of whatever liquor had the most in the bottle, into a small 2-3 ounce juice glass. I would take it and some cookies or something else sweet to chase it with back to my room and sip and nibble and fall into blissful sleep. I never drank enough during those days to experience a hangover. I didn't do it every night, usually only on weekends when I didn't have studying or school to get up for. I knew that I would not get by with this indefinitely as my parents would be sure to notice the slowly decreasing supply of alcohol. I surrounded myself with a handful of really good friends in middle school. All were male except for my best friend since birth, Tami. But Tami moved ½ hour away when I was thirteen (which might as well have been the moon because we couldn't yet drive and this was before cell phones or social media). So it was mainly me and the guys.

One of my friends had a much older sibling who would supply us/me with alcohol. For some reason, the first bottle he gave to me was brandy. This, I loved. Used mainly for sleep and not every day, a big bottle would last me forever. But I was ever vigilant regarding my supply on hand for I did not want to run out. In talking to many "normies," this behavior is not normal amongst people who drink normally. Damn those normies!

On and on, this continued. Sometimes I could only get beer, which I hate but it still did the job. I kept a case in my room disguised inside a mountain dew case, warm, and at night if I needed it, would pour one can over ice and that would be enough to help me sleep. Notice I say "needed," even then. I needed a drink—to sleep, to calm, to numb. I had found something to rely on to keep me sane and sleeping and successful. It worked! My high school career soared. I was homecoming queen, president of the student body, class valedictorian, and won a leadership scholarship to a small Christian based college four hours from home. I became an accomplished pianist, and taught lessons for several years during high school. I was doing it! I was pleasing my parents and the community and myself. Because of my successes, I also found myself a victim of haters and jealousy, which at the time I could not understand. I was not being mean, I was not bullying; I was being kind and trying to fit in. I was good at almost everything I tried, and that is hard for other teenagers to handle sometimes. Now, looking back, I can see how this might have been to some of those who didn't like me. Akin to the question of whether anyone in the country actually wants the New England Patriots to make it to another Super Bowl (give somebody else a chance for once!!!), though on a much lesser scale. As yummy as Tom Brady and Gronk are to watch, it would be nice to see some other teams succeed. Although my handful of tried and true guy friends remained stable, I never did again find a female friend besides Tami that I felt I could trust until I became sober. They were there all along, but my walls were already going up, my need to not be vulnerable, and my desire to be seen as untouchable and perfect. I was pretentious as could be and did not realize it.

During the summers of my high school years, I lived mostly independently at our lake cabin. I worked two jobs, maintenance at a resort and cooking at a small café/grocery store. My family would come on the weekends, but during the week, that solitude I craved was all mine. I would swim and sunbathe, bake, and even played piano at a small church just down the road. I worked hard and earned a lot of money, while being away from the day-to-day pressures I felt at home. My drinking continued as well, but did not increase on a daily level, surprisingly. I had too much going for me, too much to lose, to get in trouble or disappoint anyone. It was at this time that alcohol again compromised my morals. I had stolen alcohol from my parents, yes, but that did not feel like a major breach of morality to me. However, while working at the grocery store during the summers, and away from my normal booze supplier, I resorted to stealing beer. Beer, because that's the only alcohol the grocery store sold. I wasn't old enough to buy it, so I felt I had no other recourse. I justified and rationalized constantly. Again, a case of beer would typically last me twenty-four days, so the amount I was stealing didn't amount to much of a loss for the store—at least that's what I told myself to calm my guilt. I also began experimenting more with larger amounts of alcohol when my guy friends would join me and bring more.

During one of those summers, with the same cousin whom I had enjoyed that first champagne fountain, I attended a sketchy party. We all had too much to drink, and wanting to get out of there before any trouble started, we left, with me behind the wheel. On a dark gravel road, with my cousin and another girl in the car, I lost control and we spun several times around before landing right side up in the ditch. None of us were wearing seat belts, nobody did in those days, plus we were too cool for that. Remarkably, we were able to drive right out and get home safely. It was a bit of a rough and lopsided ride home, but we made it. The flat tire on my car was explained away to my parents with an "I don't know what happened." They bought it. And so, the driving drunk had begun. Another line I had been determined not to cross, had been run right over. I got away with it and should have learned my lesson. But of course, I had not.

My guy friends continued to be a constant, despite my dating several other boys during high school. I adored them, and they adored me. And I liked it like that. I was seeking love, adoration, support, and friendship. I felt validated because these friends loved me. But they all also were attracted to me. I knew that, and I liked that because it boosted my awful self-esteem. The four of us, the three boys and me, had a lot of fun. One of them had parents who were often away on extended vacations, leaving him alone in a glorious home with beautiful lush indoor gardens, gorgeous furnishings, and a wine cellar. One night, when his parents were gone, the boys cooked a tasty steak dinner and we imbibed on several bottles of wine. I played piano for them, albeit sloppily I am sure, yet I felt proud and happy. Ever persistent was my need not to disappoint my parents, I could not fathom calling them to say I was in no shape to drive home. So, after spending an hour or so in the bathroom violently sick from too much wine, I drove home. I took the back roads and had to stop every five minutes with the dry heaves. I made it home safely, and nobody at home was ever the wiser. I got by with it again. Man, I was so smart and sneaky. This was too easy! What could ever go wrong? I was unbalanced, to a spectacular degree. But it took me years to realize. I was a scared little girl trying to be perfect for everyone, putting on this show—this shell— for everyone to see, while inside I was becoming less and less like that girl and my true substance was dissipating. A dual life was being led. And that, my friends, is a lot of work to maintain.

ᴄ♪Chapter Threeᴏᴠᴏ

The College Years

ttending a Christian college while being a heavy drinker only furthered the divide between my façade and reality. In order to maintain my scholarship, I was required to participate in a multitude of extracurricular and leadership activities. This included music, student council, and a coveted role in a Christian traveling theater troop. Within this group of twelve were some of the most kind, faithful, and truly good people. One has gone on to travel the world with Habitat for Humanity, while spreading the word of God. Another has used his musical talents to write, record, and perform his music across the country bringing the message of God to everyone he can. One has become a youth pastor. Our director retired from his position and went on to become an upstanding politician, fighting for his Christian beliefs. On and on, their stories then and their stories now are the textbook examples of human perfection. No one in the group drank, except for me. Everyone in the group, besides me, was a virgin. These people were better than me, I believed. This is what being a good person should look like, and I came into the group already, in my opinion, mortally flawed. Yet, I faked it. I didn't fake my belief in God or my individual spirituality, though I was continuing to lead this double life. I pretended like I belonged there, though in my heart, I didn't believe I deserved it. And to numb this nagging and worsening feeling of inadequacy, I drank. Still not daily, still not during the day, but at night to make those horrid thoughts of self-loathing abate, albeit temporarily. At least I could sleep.

I intended to major in science, as I desired a career in medicine. I wanted a lucrative career, yet one in which I could help people. The majority of others at this college were majoring in parochial education. They all wanted to be church schoolteachers! Isn't that hilarious?? What was I doing there? They were all so sound and solid in their faith and their convictions, their morality and ethics seemingly concrete. I did not fit in with this crowd, though I did a bang up job of making it look like I did. I believed in God, had attended church and been confirmed, and participated in every church music performance possible during my primary and secondary education. But, in looking back, my motives for that participation were not authentic. It was a way to continue to showcase my talents, receive accolades, and observe as my parents beamed with pride over those accomplishments. I wasn't participating to honor or glorify God. I was participating to honor and glorify myself. That was a revolting discovery to make about myself later in life, when I finally became sober and could see my past for what it really was.

Some of my classmates in college, like at any college I assume, were beginning to test their independence and try out the wilder things in life, including drinking. Many of them never did, but those that did often drank to excess and got sick and in trouble and I wanted no part of that. Going to a party at the neighboring U of M with a bunch of strangers and drugs and who knows what was not in my wheelhouse. No thank you. I was perfectly happy to keep my bottle under my bed and imbibe alone. As expected, I quickly found a twenty-one- year old male classmate who would happily buy my brandy for me. At least this time I was giving him money and not just stealing it from the store! I continued to experience success. Excellent grades, maintained my scholarship, participated in theater rehearsals and performances including fantastic trips to Venezuela, NYC, Germany, and even a performance in front of thousands of teenagers at a national youth gathering. I took on part time jobs including work at a convenience store and working ten pm to 2 am shifts at a group home for disabled adults. Again, my motives were not altogether altruistic—I was doing this to pad my resume as by that time, I was looking forward to graduate school to become a Physician Assistant.

I was then given the amazing opportunity to play piano at a prestigious club in downtown St. Paul. It paid an incredible amount of money for a college student, with the bonus that I got to dress up in fancy dresses and heels four nights a week. This, I loved. Often I would be tipped with cash or glasses of wine for requested songs. One gentleman, a self-made multi-millionaire immigrant from Lebanon, whose name is on buildings all over St. Paul, would tip me fifty bucks each time he came in if I played his favorite song. I happened to know it the first time he asked, a Spanish tune called "Maleguena," and after that first time, it was a given. If I played it, he gave me a crisp fifty. This created a soaring boost of self-importance. And also catapulted me into what I thought was an adult life. Fancy dresses, big money, self-reliance, tit for tat.

By that time, my own need for success and accolades had surpassed my need to please my parents, though not replaced. I began applying to PA schools. My first choices were the #1 and #2 schools in the country, Duke and the University of Iowa. The U of I invited me for an interview and I was accepted. First round of interviews. I was elated. Duke never did invite me for an interview, but I didn't tell anyone that. I just told everyone I got accepted to my first choice. I couldn't deal with rejection, even in the face of acceptance by another entity. I was so dysfunctional. Yet functioning and succeeding, at least on the outside.

I became good friends with two of the rare other science majors, who were both also planning on medical careers—one in physical therapy and another PA school like me. We studied medical vocabulary, chemistry, and biology together. Late nights at Applebee's eating half price apps and drinking soda studying for exams became a regular occurrence. These two young women were, and still are, amazing and solid Christian women. They were not drinkers, they were not partying, they were not having sex, and they attended chapel every day. I looked like I did the same, except for the chapel thing because everybody knew I didn't like to get up early. I kept my drinking and affairs and other life well hidden. Yet I found friendship in these two women. I feared that if they knew who I really was, deep inside, my sins and past and all, that they wouldn't like me anymore. I began to have that fear about a lot of people during this time. I mention these two in particular, because they are amazing women. I just wish I would have, could have let them in back then. I isolated myself from near certain true and lasting friendships for one reason. I drank. And with drinking came poor decisions resulting in shame, and with shame came fear of discovery.

I let my roommate in a bit more probably out of pure proximity, despite that she is truly a genuine and selfless person. She was studying to become a parochial school teacher. She was the RA on our floor. She knew I drank and didn't flinch at me keeping it in the room. I wasn't causing any trouble, wasn't getting obviously drunk, just minded my own business. She would drink occasionally, but very rarely. She had a boyfriend that she began dating at age fourteen. They are married and still together to this day, having had two biological children and adopted two less fortunate children. I was trying to live up to this woman who seemed perfect to me. I wasn't good enough to be in her presence, but I tried to act like I was. I think I was afraid of "good people" like her, because I didn't feel I measured up. I was so afraid of being found out for the fraud I really was. Fear had taken a near permanent seat driving my life.

✑Chapter Four✑

GRADUATE SCHOOL

I was in!! I made it. I was accepted. Out of over 600 applicants, twenty-three were accepted for spots in the Masters Degree Program for Physician Assistant Studies, and I was one of them. I was elated. My future looked bright and there was no stopping me now. Within this class, were people that were married with kids, divorced, married without kids, single, young, older, from all walks of life. It was the University of Iowa, a large campus in the awesome college town of Iowa City. This was not the small religious college I had previously attended. These people were real, with pasts, imperfect like me. There was no chapel service every morning, no quaint discussions about spirituality, no pressure to be perfect. Everyone drank to relax and reward after big study sessions or stressful exams. The whole city drank, it seemed. Here, I fit in. Exams and grades were pass or fail, no worries about obtaining straight A's. The person in the class who graduated with the lowest GPA was still going to be called a PA! Finally! I could be myself.

PA training was hard. HARD! It was most challenging thing I have ever done in my life, up until getting sober, which was both harder and more rewarding. The training was grueling. We took a year of courses with a couple hundred second year medical students. We dissected human cadavers. We studied, we learned, we stressed. We drank together. We had a year of clinical rotations which often required ridiculous hours and little sleep. We had study groups. We went out for dinner and more drinks. We prepared and presented our individual research projects. We supported each other and there was minimal competition which was so refreshing. And all but one of us became PA's. We became a close knit group, many paired up into dating couples. In fact, two sets of couples from that small group eventually married. I was one of them.

Enter Jim. I was struggling with biochemistry. Jim and I had a common connection being Minnesota natives educating in Iowa. Jim had recently completed graduate level courses in biochemistry at the U of M, and had it down pat. He became my tutor, for lack of better terminology. We met often, at late night diners, him helping me to grasp the concepts, us learning about each other in the process. We studied our other courses together as well, and I passed biochemistry with his help.

Jim and I drank together. People who abuse substances often surround themselves with others who use and abuse the same substances equally or even those that use more than they do. It is a defense mechanism that helps us to be able to compare and say "well, he drinks as much as I do so I am fine," or "she drinks more than I do, and she is successful, so I don't have a problem." This was very dangerous for me, for both of us. We rewarded our hard work and successes with heavy drinking. I engaged in risky drunk driving frequently. Uber was not around, cabs were few and far between and expensive. We were poor and starving graduate students, so money was not free flowing. At least those were among the many excuses I used to rationalize my behavior.

Jim was married. We became more than friends. We were best friends. We were attracted to each other. Many diary entries from that time reveal my angst that I was attracted to this man though I should not be. He felt the same. His marriage was not perfect, they argued a great deal, and Jim was not happy. However, me entering the equation elevated his dissatisfaction within his marriage. I listened and agreed with him about any negative thing he had to say about his wife and his marriage. We continued to see each other daily, study hard, drink hard, and fell into an alcohol infused love. Eventually, one night after way too much liquor, we crossed the line. We slept together. We felt horrible guilt, and both insisted it would never happen again. It did. I was madly in love with this unavailable man. Instead of walking away, I continued with it. I craved love so badly and always had. From the start, craving my daddy's love and affection and approval, I had been quite male dependent. I needed that attention for my self-esteem. I didn't want to be single, for that must mean something was wrong with me. But, I often chose men who were not good for me, who were unavailable, who I didn't really love or have much in common with, and men who were abusive in one way or another. And I tended to go from one relationship right into the next, never allowing myself to be alone or learn who I really was; never learning to be comfortable without a relationship. But, when I tired of a relationship, I was quick to break hearts and move on. In this case, we truly did love each other. I was head over heels and was certain he was "the one." We had so much in common and had such ease in conversations. He was so funny, and often the life of the party. When we were out, he typically drank more than me and was much more loud spoken, therefore my drinking tended to be less noticeable to others, which I liked. He was confident—almost arrogant, handsome, smart, and a take-charge kind of guy. Some of the same traits my dad had. Just what I needed, because it was comfortable for me to become what he needed me to be and follow his lead. But we both abused alcohol, he was married, and I was a master in codependence. We were a recipe for explosions and disaster if we continued on that way. Yet we did.

Chapter Five

MARRIED LIFE

Jim had divorced his wife. We moved in together and began our careers and life as a couple. It wasn't long, and we became engaged. The marriage proposal was epic. EPIC! Disneyworld had always been, and still is, one of my favorite places on earth. My family had a timeshare in Orlando, so we went almost every year. However, I had never stayed in one of the resort hotels. We went with my sister and her then boyfriend/now husband to the Magic Kingdom. At the end of the day, Jim surprised me having brought an overnight bag and keys to stay at the Contemporary Resort, overlooking the Magic Kingdom. I had no idea he had already saved enough money for a ring and was convinced that the hotel stay (not inexpensive), was my Christmas gift, as this was around the Christmas holiday, December 29th to be exact. He had asked my father for permission and Dad had given it. My parents and sister were all cautious regarding Jim, considering the circumstances under which we became involved. I wanted desperately to prove them wrong. The finalized divorce helped a great deal.

That evening, checked into the magic kingdom and drinking brandy on the balcony, it was about time for the fireworks. Jim got down on one knee, presented a small glass slipper with a ring in it, and asked me to marry him. I said "yes" just as the fireworks began over Cinderella's magical castle. I couldn't have been happier. Jim was like this. Friends and family were impressed with his thoughtfulness and the grandeur of such instances. Throughout our married life he would do this every couple of years—a grand piano one time in front of his entire family. He planned and executed romantic grand getaways to Boca Grande, Charleston, Kiawah Island and many other places. He even surprised me with plane tickets to see Jerry Lee Lewis, my favorite. When the concert was cancelled at the last minute, even though we were already at the destination, he took me to dinners and plays and then redid the whole vacation in a month for the rescheduled concert. We were successful in our careers, financially well ahead of our peers, and wanted to start a family. We had a miscarriage with our first pregnancy, at sixteen weeks. We had not told our family or friends that we were pregnant yet. I felt shame, I felt that I had somehow caused or deserved it, so much so that we never told our families about it until several months later when I required emergency surgery due to an incomplete miscarriage. I dealt with the loss on my own, and stuffed my emotions with alcohol. We were blessed to go on to have two beautiful children, Tate and Olivia, after the miscarriage. I somehow white knuckled it sober through the pregnancies and Jim cut down. However, when our bag was packed for each baby arrival, along with tiny outfits and diapers, was liquor. We celebrated each delivery almost immediately with booze. Who does that? But, from the outside looking in, things appeared perfect. This is how I wanted it.

But inside, there was trouble. Our daily drinking continued. Drinks right after work. Drinking at home together into every late night, until I passed out. Yet, we continued to do well in our jobs, both quite functional. We were not daytime drinkers, except occasionally on weekends if we had friends over for boating or lake life. We introduced liquor into all holiday gatherings among my extended family. His family always had events centered around alcohol. Parties, reunions, weddings, even funerals in his family included copious amounts of alcohol consumed by nearly everyone.

I tended to be a happy and quiet drunk, sometimes funny, but mostly to drink until I was numb and forget reality. Jim, on the other hand, was an angry drunk. The first few drinks, he was funny—delightful in fact. After that, he could become angry, irritated, dominated conversations, and just wasn't fun for people to be around, including me.

On our honeymoon, for example, we obviously drank heavily. We were in Reno the first night prior to going to Lake Tahoe to spend the rest of our vacation. Late at night, drunk, we ordered room service. I passed out. As I recall it, when room service arrived, I was too tired to eat it. He became so angry about this that he threw the food and plates and glassware all around the room. It was frightening. I took a pillow and blanket and locked myself in the bathroom to spend my first night of our honeymoon. I heard him finally leave the room, and I grabbed my suitcase and went out to the rental car, contemplating returning home. What stopped me was the fact that I didn't want my family or friends to have been right. I wanted our marriage to work, more for the benefit of appearances than I like to admit, even now. But then, I didn't see it that way. I saw that my parents had just spent a lot of money on a huge wedding. I recalled them being concerned about my involvement with Jim from the start. I didn't want them to be right. So I stayed. Instances like this were frequent. Usually, I cowered and said whatever he wanted to hear. Many times, I would fight back verbally or even physically. But, Jim was an expert at arguing, and I could never win, so I typically withdrew and refused to talk to him or engage with him for days in classic passive-aggressive form. Or, I apologized. Even the many times I felt that I had totally been in the right; again an impressive example of my covert manipulation—not saying how I felt, not putting my foot down. And certainly not recommending we quit drinking.

On another specific occasion, we had taken our kids—then two and four boating over to a local restaurant. We both were drinking, and Jim became loud and obnoxious, the way I saw it anyway. He later admitted he had been drinking all day due to some major stress he was feeling at work. I asked him to try to tone it down because other patrons, some of whom we knew, were noticing and looking at us. Of course, I wanted us to look perfect, so this spectacle made me uncomfortable and angry. I went out of my way to be inconspicuous, and Jim loved the spotlight. The very things that had attracted me to Jim in the beginning, were now traits that I resented. When an acquaintance came to our table and said something like "wow Jim, it sounds like you are having a great time. I can hear you all the way over at my table," that was the last straw for both of us. I ordered the waitress to box up our food that had just arrived. We got on the boat, the kids tucked in each under one of my arms, with Jim driving the boat. He gunned it, our daughter fell over. I scrambled to pick her up, he kept going, full speed all the while screaming at me. He then took each of the four to-go containers and threw them at my face, the contents flying everywhere, hitting me, the kids, the water. I made a decision that if I could; I was going to get the kids and myself out of there. He pulled the boat right up on the beach. I had my purse, which held my cell phone and keys. I grabbed the kids to attempt to get them and myself to the car. He could see what I was planning, and he punched out a window and grabbed our son. I chased him into the house and hit him with my purse until he let go of the boy. The three of us got to the car, none of us with shoes, covered in ketchup and now Jim's blood from the window, and raced away. I called my sister and asked if we could come to her house. Her husband had the sheriff waiting at the county line in the event Jim tried to follow us. My sister and her husband tried to convince me to divorce him and file charges. They told me if we didn't attend counseling at least, they would report him to the authorities and to the MN Board of Medical Practice. I didn't want that. I wasn't ready to give up. So I promised to go to counseling. Jim refused to go so I went alone. The counselor told me Jim had to quit drinking and recommended I do the same. I never went back.

We tried, on several occasions, to stop drinking. We would get it out of the house, and then one or the other of us would bring it back in. We vowed not to drink but then one of us would go out to a bar and come home with liquor on our breath and it was game on again. We then decided that all of our problems were because of his stressful job. So we moved closer to his family, much farther away from mine. Thus, began the social isolation for me. And, it should be no surprise, because we took ourselves and our booze with us when we moved, our problems did not go away.

In the new city, Jim was still unhappy in his work. I enjoyed my new position, though I had left one where they had actually built a small clinic for me to practice in a small town which was, truly, my dream job. But, my marriage was important. I wanted to keep our family together. I wanted it peaceful, I wanted Jim happy, and I still was convinced that it was my job to see to his happiness. If I was just prettier, thinner, didn't nag, whatever—I would do it. I would continue to apologize for things I did not feel were my fault, to keep the peace. I would put him to bed "the nice way" just to find some peace by myself at night where I would drink myself into a pass-out state. I began to see a counselor to try to help do better. My counselor labeled me a "peace whore." I would do anything at all to attempt to maintain the peace, except quit drinking. I wasn't the problem with drinking, Jim was. I was drinking to calm the stress and nerves of this tumultuous relationship. Isn't that what anybody in my position would do? Oh, I rationalized and justified and was always able to use him as the scapegoat because he drank more, he became angry, he was unhappy—so on and so forth.

Jim became even more unhappy. He didn't feel he was being paid well in his new position. Didn't feel he was being utilized to his fullest potential. Began to feel more worthless and unimportant which was horrible for his already tanked self-esteem. So, he drank more. We both did. He became worried that if I went out with a colleague of either sex, that I would cheat on him. If I went shopping and got home after he did, he was suspicious and angry. He began to criticize what I wore, too sexy, too revealing, too this, too that. He began to attempt to control me more, and trying to keep things calm, I became more isolated. I stopped inviting people over. I stopped doing things with colleagues. I did not make many friends or begin a new social circle. And I saw my sister and parents less and less frequently. I told him anything I thought he wanted to hear. I tried anything to make things better.

I was lonely. A slow burn of resentment had begun to simmer within me. He had taken me away from family and now was attempting to control and isolate me. I had gone along with it and supported it. I was lying to him about my true feelings. In fact, at that time I don't believe I even knew my true feelings anymore. I had lost myself. I had given control to someone—my husband, he did not take that from me. I handed it over and it became the status quo. One of the few people that were invited into our home was Jim's boss, Michael. He was a spine surgeon whom Jim had known back at the U of M during undergraduate studies and thought he was awesome. He quickly took a liking to me and it was clear he was interested beyond a friend level. I was so lonely, and angry, and by then very deep into by daily reliance of alcohol to the point of passing out every night and being hungover every morning. Decision making abilities for me at that time were poor, to say the least.

We began an affair. I had never once during our relationship cheated on Jim or considered it. But this man gave me attention. He said he loved me. He was married, too, with three girls. He said he was going to get a divorce. He said that he wanted to marry me. He wanted us to have a child together, he said. I had always strongly desired another child probably to try to fill the whole of loneliness that I felt in my heart. I already had two beautiful children, but I wanted another. Jim, at the time, did not. He was adamantly opposed to another child. Michael was a different story, or so he told me.

Chapter Six

Divorce #1

Jim discovered our affair. He was distraught and angry and terrified of losing me. By that point, I was ready to be done with our marriage. I made him leave and hired a nasty high priced attorney who loved to fight. Jim, by nature being a fighter, fought back. I threw alcoholism at him. He threw it back. We went through a custody evaluation, and the custody evaluator told us we both needed to quit drinking. Of course, we both decided not to use her findings at all during the court hearing. Neither one of us could face the fact that alcohol had any part in destroying our lives.

The divorce and custody battle became long and drawn out and lasted nearly two years, costing us over $35,000 dollars. I wanted full custody and believed I deserved it. He wanted 50/50 and believed he deserved it. The kids did not like angry drunk dad, and made that clear to the custody evaluator. However, they also did not like sad and sleeping mommy who always put on movie after movie to keep them occupied. But, that was easier to tolerate than unpredictable outbursts that were possible with their dad. I used this to my advantage and sought the services of a guardian ad litem, with the intention of helping me keep the kids safe. Little did I know how true that would become down the road in keeping them safe from me. Throughout the first portion of the separation and divorce proceedings, we both continued to work. I continued to see Michael, and although he never did leave his wife, he moved a bunch of his things into my home and lived/stayed with us whenever he could sneak away from his "real" family. I was his dirty little secret. I never met his daughters. His wife to this day does not know about our three and a half year affair, and he did not divorce her until years later.

The secret factor of my relationship with Michael simply isolated me further. I did not know when or if he would come around. I was not a part of his family or friend circle, though I had introduced him to mine. My family and friends disliked him and the situation greatly, but they all tried to be supportive. They wanted to see me happy. I would put the kids to bed, wait for him to possibly show up, get drunker and drunker, and pass out. Sometimes he would sneak into the house in the middle of the night, sometimes he would not. We went on several awesome vacations to the Bahamas, Panama, and Belize though I do not remember Belize at all except for tiny snippets because my drinking had become so advanced by that point. We had some good times, but for the most part it was a completely dysfunctional union built upon lies and cheating and fueled by my alcoholism and horrible self-esteem which convinced me I didn't deserve anything better.

On February 12, 2012, my dear cousin Jackie ended her life. I believe she struggled with her alcohol use, though I am unaware how deeply. Her death nearly destroyed her parents and her brothers, and so many of us were left feeling confused, angry, blaming ourselves or others. What did we miss? Why didn't we do this? Why didn't we do that? So many unanswered questions. Her death resonated with me on a deep and personal level. However, probably because I was so incredibly broken at the time due to my own alcoholism, loneliness, and anxiety, her suicide hit very close to home. I could totally understand why she might have made that decision. I was beginning to know the hopelessness, the desperation, and the dark and scary places in the recesses of my mind that I just had to saturate with the drink to numb. Both her family service and funeral were so well attended that the church was bursting at the seams. This vibrant, funny, gentle, and kind-hearted woman had touched so many lives and had so many people who loved her, yet she had finally found it unbearably painful to continue in life. Once again, alcohol was my friend to help me deal with that tragedy. Her suicide could and should have scared me straight, but instead, I only progressed further into a downward spiral.

Shortly after that my ex, Jim got a gross misdemeanor DWI. He was fired from his job. He was unable to pass his PA recertification boards and was unable to get a different job without that certification. Instead of treating him with compassion and grace, I used this to my advantage, got the guardian involved, and was awarded sole physical custody with Jim having visitation awarded a few hours a week. During the hearing, he brought up my drinking but I denied any problems. We both went through chemical dependency evaluations, I lied my way through mine and had Michael and my sister lie for me to corroborate my story. I wanted the kids with me, and truly believed at the time that they were better off with me. I did not see that I was using them as emotional support and to not be alone. They slept with me in my bedroom. I pacified them with delivery pizza and movies while I slept and drank and drank some more and slept some more. Looking back, the neglect I was inflicting upon my beautiful children is sickening. I have worked very hard in sobriety to deal with the guilt and shame incurred because of that. If you are not an alcoholic, you are probably detesting my behavior and having difficulty understanding it. If you are an alcoholic you are perhaps nodding. I couldn't understand how my drinking was affecting the kids and didn't even see that it was hurting them. In fact my brain at the time had me convinced that I was still a great mom. It was insanity.

One night, when Jim came to the house to bring the kids home, he pushed his way past me into the house, went to the liquor cabinet which was stocked and took pictures and video with his phone. I was terrified. From that day forward, I did my drinking much more secretively. I moved the liquor into my bedroom walk in closet and did most of my drinking from there, straight out of the bottles. As anyone who has ever hidden alcohol knows, when the hiding and drinking secretly begins, things often go to hell in a hurry. I wanted to drink, but knew the kids were old enough to tell their dad and/or the guardian if they saw me drinking. So, I would run to the closet frequently, slam down a few gulps, and return as if nothing was amiss. I was always unsure how long it would be before I got back to the closet, so I drank more each time than I probably would have if it had been in a glass like a normal person out in the open. I also had to remedy the situation of having the only drinking spot being the closet. I began hiding bottles in the laundry room, under the sink in my bathroom, in the upstairs bathroom, in the linen closet, in the basket of blankets in the living room, in the garage—anywhere I didn't think the kids would look but where I could easily get to it if needed. But never in the open for fear of being discovered. At this point, a normal person would have just stopped drinking for the sake of the kids. It seems so obvious and completely crazy not to. But I was not normal. I was an alcoholic. I put alcohol above everything sacred in my life. Alcohol had become my master. And a brutal master it was.

❦Chapter Seven❧

Detox #1

My divorce was finalized. I was still seeing Michael. I had the kids. I had my work. I was still, somehow, seeing patients every day, hungover all morning. I would chew gum and use hand sanitizer in front of each patient, in the event that they smelled alcohol, I hoped they would assume it was the hand sanitizer. I never drank in the morning or during work, until I did.

I began running home for "lunch." I would have a couple shots of vodka. As any good alcoholic knows, vodka has the reputation for being the least detectable odor-wise on the breath. After getting by with this for a while, I started also drinking a few shots first thing in the morning before work to get myself going and calm the shakes and nausea. Sometimes, I would vomit immediately. As soon as the heaves stopped, I would attempt to swig again. It wasn't until I got some vodka to stay inside me, that I began to feel semi-normal. After a while, four hours between drinks was too much. I started filling a water bottle with vodka and sipping it at my desk. Amazingly, my charts always were competed, my documentation sound, my patients happy (as evidenced by the stellar patient satisfaction results I still obtained), and I never hurt anybody. No one at work ever called me out on suspicion, no patients ever reported me, and the entire workplace was legitimately surprised to learn of my alcoholism.

Michael was still coming around on his terms, I was feeling more and more like a dirty secret. I had even tried dating someone else, but Michael was persistent. He actually took my phone one night when I was passed out and texted the gentleman I had been seeing, texting him all sorts of nasty messages. He deleted the messages. Of course I found out about this. I tried to smooth things over with both men, and for some unknown reason, probably because I didn't feel worthy enough of the other man, I went back to Michael. I was so lonely and sad, and was veering further away from the person I wanted to be with each passing day. The guilt, the shame, the cravings, and the withdrawal were catching up with me. Thoughts of suicide became frequent. My sister and her husband convinced me to call things off with Michael, my best friend Tami agreed. Everyone believed him and our situation was not good for me. So I did. But I was so lonely.

One particularly awful night after far too much to drink, in and out of consciousness, I called my sister who was in Chicago on business. I don't know what I said to her. I am sure it wasn't all roses and kindness and I am not sure she could even understand me. But, she knew things were not right. She also knew the kids were with me. She took the next flight to Minneapolis, rented a car, and drove straight to me. Apparently, she found me in between incoherent and passed out. The kids were scared and hungry and lonely. She called my parents, who made the five hour drive in record time. My father, whom I still so desperately wanted approval from, came to my bedroom. I was, by then, able to talk. I bawled and hugged him and asked if he still loved me. He assured me he did. He asked what in the world were we going to do. I told him I needed to go to detox. He took me to Fairview Riverside in Minneapolis. They miraculously had an opening. I blew a .321 and had not had a drink for a couple of hours before the testing. My father later told me he thought I was going to die in his car on the way there. When registering, which I barely recall, they handed me a sheet asking me what I was there for and I shakily chicken scratched out the word DETOX. Dad stayed with me while they ordered tests and gave me fluids infused with vitamins and Ativan to calm the withdrawal and prevent seizures that can go along with alcohol withdrawal. My labs confirmed alcoholic ketoacidosis and my liver enzymes were three times the normal levels. I was stabilized and admitted to the detox floor. I was so hopeful that if I could just get help to stop, that I could then stay stopped and get back to my normal life. I was sure this was all situational—the divorce, the relationship with Michael, the custody battle, my cousin

Jackie's suicide. I just drank to cope. I did not believe I was an alcoholic.

I was feeling better because of the fluids and Ativan. I was admitted to the locked detox floor where they did a strip search, took my belongings, cut the strings off sweatshirts and pants to minimize the risk I may use those strings to kill myself, and basically made me feel like a criminal. The rooms were double rooms and the doors to the bathrooms were only partial doors, so that staff could always get in if needed. It seemed like jail. There were no mirrors. Makeup was not allowed. Showers had a small button that provided about a thirty-second squirt of water each time so you had to keep pushing the button to get a complete shower. I guess that was to decrease the risk of someone attempting to drown themselves. Phones were definitely not allowed. I did not belong there. I was feeling better and should be able to leave now. I was not going to stay there another minute. I actually thought that my kids needed me! Yes of course, they needed a drunk and unstable neglectful mom, right. They were now at home with my parents who were loving them and feeding them and giving them the attention they so badly craved and deserved. Yet, I was convinced I did not need to stay in detox any longer. However, the paperwork I had signed upon intake to detox apparently basically held me in the facility for no less than forty-eight hours. I bucked, I begged, I sobbed, I pleaded. Nope. I attempted to unlock the drawer that contained my phone with a hairpin that they had inadvertently not confiscated from me. I attempted to unlock the main door with the same hairpin. I tried to figure out how I could get out of my non-functioning fifth floor window. I am not exactly sure what I thought I was going to do if I succeeded with my escape, with no money, no phone, no keys, wearing hospital scrubs labeled "DETOX", and without shoes in December in Minnesota—but I wanted OUT.

I learned quickly from others on the unit who had been there before. They told me that forty-eight hours was the minimum stay. And that I couldn't be released until I had not required any Ativan for 24 hours and had no vomiting for twenty-four hours with stable vitals. They checked me for shakes, made me stick out my tongue and checked my vitals every couple of hours and recorded the results. If I met their numerical criteria for requiring more Ativan, it was given. I didn't want any more Ativan because I knew it would delay my release. So I tried to refuse. They let me refuse if I was below a certain number. I learned if I flexed my hands and fingers the right way I could do it without them shaking. I practiced sticking out my tongue in my reflection from the window of my room, remember there were no mirrors (which could be broken and used to cut yourself). I practiced until I could use my tongue muscles a certain way so that it did not quiver. I couldn't fake my way out of my racing pulse very well, though as a PA, I was aware that if you are inspiring your pulse goes up and upon exhale, it drops. So, when they were checking my pulse, I made sure to do a super long exhale. I started to pass the tests (correction: cheat on the tests), so that I didn't have to receive any more Ativan. I was sick, though, and would vomit frequently. Of course, I told no one. They were making me eat, of which I had done very little of recently, and the amount I ate also was scored and counted for or against my release. Once, I didn't make it to the toilet and vomited all over my room. I proceeded to rapidly clean up the room with paper towels and put the paper towels in the paper bag that was the "trash can" in the room (plastic bags were a no-no, suffocation risk) and then took the whole mess to the community trash can in the dining room (yes, yuck) so no staff was the wiser about my inability to keep food down. Whew!

The countdown to discharge from that hellhole was on. I had time to kill, though. I was forced to attend a couple of meetings. They weren't for me because I certainly did not have anything in common with those people. The other people there were seasoned in addiction. They had lost everything. Some of them were criminals. Many had lost their children. One man was served divorce papers in there. I had nothing like that. I was nothing like them. A particularly helpful patient mentioned the "Blue Book" and asked if I had a copy. I did not. I did not even know what he was referring to. He showed me a copy of his. It was the Big Book of Alcoholics Anonymous. I had no interest. I just wanted to get out of there and never, ever come back. I was nowhere near accepting that I was an alcoholic, or that I needed help. I just wanted to be let out.

Houston we have a problem. In all of my drunken honesty upon intake to detox, I had told them what I did for a living, that I was a licensed and practicing medical provider, and also that I had been drinking at work. They are mandated reporters. Whoops. Shit. So, what happens now? You know, that Ativan I had been refusing for the last forty-eight hours sure sounded pretty good right about then. They gave me the option of self-reporting my situation to an organization I had never heard of before called HPSP (Health Professional Services Program). If I didn't, they were going to report me to the MN Board of Medical Practice. Oh, my God! *Why* had I been honest? Fear and panic ensued but were replaced quickly with the decision to take the easiest route of reporting to the HPSP thing. Whatever that was, it had to be better than the Board of Medical practice getting involved. I needed a paycheck, I needed my job. I had worked so hard to be at this point in my career and was almost seventeen years into it. I did not want to lose this. I called HPSP, recorded and witnessed by my detox caseworker. I answered her questions honestly, mainly because this caseworker who already knew what I had admitted to, was sitting right there breathing down my neck. I was now enrolled in HPSP. Which turned out to be a big, big fricking deal.

Chapter Eight

HPSP

My first caseworker at HPSP, a woman named Marilyn, was very kind but firm about the requirements of this program. Basically, it is a way to monitor healthcare professionals in the state of Minnesota with addictions of one type or another, without having to get the Board of Medical Practice involved. The state wants and needs medical providers to be practicing, but the goal of these government agencies above all else is public safety. They wanted to protect my patients from my drinking. Smart.

My requirements were that I attend at least two recovery meetings a week, attend a specific health care provider recovery meeting once a month, find a therapist, find a sponsor, find a doctor, and have all of these people report to HPSP on a quarterly basis regarding my progress and whether I was maintaining sobriety. Another requirement was that I call in to a phone number every day before 4 pm. It is a color system, apparently random. My colors were to be purple and white. If either of my colors was called, I was required to submit a urine sample to test for drugs and alcohol. The newest alcohol testing, EtG, could detect even trace amounts of alcohol for the previous five to seven days. I was going to provide nine specimens a quarter, or about three times a month but random. I never would know when my color would be called. It could be three days in a row, or it could be twice in one week with nothing for the next two weeks. My enrollment was set for a three year monitoring commitment. If I satisfied these requirements, at the end of three years, my case would be closed. If, at any point, I failed a urine drug and alcohol screen or failed to submit the required paperwork, I would be reported to the Board of Medical Practice and asked to cease practice. Yikes.

I also needed to find a work site monitor. Although neither Fairview nor HPSP were going to report my situation to my current employer, it was my responsibility to find a colleague or boss to also report to HPSP quarterly regarding my work attendance and performance as well as any suspicions of use. But, HPSP was going to allow me to go right back to work as long as I complied. Prior to my release from Detox, I needed to call someone at work, tell them my situation, and ask them to be my worksite monitor. Not knowing who to call, I thought hard about the different eighty-six providers within my clinic. I recalled one who was especially good at mental health and seemed compassionate. I called him. He was extremely gracious and kind, agreed to be my work site monitor, and asked me to come to his office when I returned to work.

43

There were visiting hours one day while I was still in detox. Michael came to see me, even though I had broken things off with him. I was grateful for that. I made sure he visited at a different time than my parents. He brought me some warm socks. He spent time with me. It seemed he really loved me and wanted me to get better. Yet, he was still married and I was still his side dish. I didn't see it that way, though. I saw it as him supporting me even when I had failed, even though I was weak. I couldn't turn away his attention then. My parents visited, and because of my sobbing wreck performances, the detox staff made special allowances to let my kids, who were eight and ten, visit as well. It was so good to see them. They seemed fine. They were happy to see me and wanted me to come home and be OK. I promised them I would.

Finally I was discharged. My parents picked me up. I told them how I was feeling so much better, and detailed what HPSP was all about, and told them "I got this." I also told them that I could easily stop drinking for three years, it wasn't forever, and that I would just get through these three years and go on with my life. They were quite skeptical. I was talking fast, trying to convince them as well as myself that what I was saying was actually true. Aside from drying out for a couple of days, I hadn't accepted or learned a damn thing. My girlfriend Maureen, who had been supportive throughout this whole ordeal, came over and all of us somewhat ceremoniously dumped all remaining liquor down the drain.

Upon returning to work the next day, I went to the office of my new worksite monitor. He told me to shut the door and sit down. He told me "Karla, I don't know why you chose me, but I have sixteen years sobriety and I understand what you are going through." I was floored but relieved. Someone else who had struggled was successfully practicing and doing well! What a relief!

I received my enrollment letter from HPSP, which stated that I officially started my program with them and was required to start calling in and submitting samples in about a month. A whole month to wait for the safety of accountability with serious consequences for failure— hmm. A trip to Disneyworld with my sister and her family, my parents, my kids and I had been long planned to take place over the Christmas holiday. My parents encouraged me to cancel this trip and just stay home and focus on sobriety, work, and the kids. But the kids and cousins were excited about this trip. I wanted everything "back to normal" so I insisted that I would be fine and still planned to go. My parents went back to their home five hours away to prepare for the trip. It was indeed back to normal, just me and my kids, school and work, day in day out. I was trying to compensate for my past bad behavior by being the best mom I could. I was so anxious and irritable, having full blown panic attacks and episodes of sobbing for no apparent reason. I was certainly not doing a good job being a mother. I couldn't cope without drinking but I could not figure out why. I began to think I was flawed, to the point of no return.

Returning to work was stressful, though, and I no longer had my crutch of booze to get me through. The same stressors and pressures and pace were there, yet I had no idea how to handle all of that without drinking. I lasted eight days before I began drinking again. I made deals with myself: only after work, only two drinks. Only brandy, no more vodka. With a land speed record, I broke every one of those deals. I couldn't eat. I couldn't sleep. I remember wandering around the house in the middle of the night lying down in each of the six beds to see if I could sleep there. But I could not. I would drink, try to drink some PowerAde, vomit everything up. At my bedside I always had vodka, PowerAde, and a puke bucket.

By the time the trip arrived, I had passed the level of illness I had been at prior to detox. The morning we were to leave for the airport, I was sluggishly moving around the house packing things while drinking vodka out of hidden bottles stashed everywhere. We got in the car. I got lost on the way to the airport—a trip I had successfully made countless times before. What was wrong with me?

We made it safely to the airport on time, thank God. By the gate was a bar. I ordered smoothies for the kids and straight vodka for myself. We were then seated in the back row of the plane. Those seats don't recline. I desperately needed to sleep. Attempting to lie down on the floor in front of our seats, I was quickly reprimanded by the flight attendants. Lying on the floor of a commercial airplane en-route was apparently not OK. Who knew?

Following a successful landing, retrieval of bags, and obtaining a rental car, we drove out into the sunlight of Florida in December. I could not, for the life of me, remember how to get to the resort that we had stayed in a dozen times in my life. I drove about aimlessly. I stopped at a couple of gas stations to ask for directions. I stopped at a liquor store and picked up a small bottle of vodka, because I needed it for this drive. Here it was, morning, and I was driving around Florida drunk, with an open container, and my babies in the backseat. The insanity of it all was, and still is, shocking. It was too stressful. Finally, distraught and confused, I had my ten- year-old son call my dad. He guided us onto the right highway and we finally made it to our destination. We stopped at the local Walmart for some groceries, as well as the local liquor store for a big bottle of brandy and got ourselves checked into our suite. We were the first of our family to arrive. My sister and her family would be coming later that night, and my parents the next day. The three of us spent the day at the pool. I was, of course, drinking the entire time. We actually had a pretty good time, I think, though my recollection is quite hazy.

Evening came, we ordered pizza, and I put the kids to bed in their room. I continued to drink heavily. I called my friend Tami, and did the whole drunk talk thing with her where I guess I mumbled and talked in circles and she became concerned and somehow got me off the phone. She called my sister, who by that point, was in the air. I crawled into my bed after drinking to the point of passing out.

Loud door banging that went on for seemingly hours woke me. I kept hoping that whoever it was would just go away. They did not. The banging got louder and more insistent. The way I recall it in my drunken haze, is that I stumbled my way to the door and opened it to find my sister, who was armed with the heads up she had received via voicemail from Tami. She barged right in past me, asked where the kids were. For some reason, I responded with "I thought they were with you." Um, no. They were in bed, I had put them there. She was, understandably concerned and frightened and furious. She said she was going to take them for the night. I argued with her. Before long, the kids were awake due to the commotion, and came out to see what was going on. My sister called her husband to come over as well. While her husband stood back and she threatened to take the kids so I could sleep it off, I started to physically attack her and try to push her out of the room. She fought back. It involved slapping and scratching, punching and clothes ripping—all in front of my kids. She was sober and strong, I was drunk and weak, yet I put up a pretty good fight. In hindsight, it was mainly because she was threatening my ability to drink. She attempted to call the police. I am not sure what ended up happening there because the police never arrived, and she and her husband ended up leaving. I locked the doors and took the kids with me into the master bathroom where we hid for a while. I told the kids that my sister was trying to take them away from me. Since she periodically could be heard pounding on the door and yelling, they

48

believed me, and they were scared. We were up almost all night in that tiny bathroom.

I knew we couldn't stay there. My life as I knew it was being threatened and I wouldn't have it. Early the next morning, with all bags packed and a plan to secretly drive over to Clearwater and have our vacation there, we were walking out the door. There, in our path, was my sister and her husband, as well as my aunt. Oh boy. My aunt had lost her daughter, my beautiful cousin Jackie, to suicide, only a few months prior. Her tears, her persuasion that she couldn't go through losing someone else, brought my defenses down. The jig was up.

The three of them convinced me that inpatient treatment was necessary. My brother in law told me he would pay for the whole thing. I made excuses, but each one was easily handled by one of my three interventionists. Calls were made to Hazelden back in Minnesota, and I completed the entire intake. The facility was full, there was a waiting list, and besides I was out of state. But, the wheels were in motion. My brother in law poured all of my liquor down the drain. The counselor at Hazelden warned my sister that abrupt cessation of drinking could lead to seizures and recommended they either take me to an ER, or allow me to drink small amounts frequently. My sister was not at all comfortable with me continuing to drink, and I was not at all comfortable with going to the ER. I had some Xanax tablets with me, and the counselor assured my sister that would prevent the seizures.

We all sobbed, and talked, and hugged, and discussed treatment. I was resigned to it, at that moment anyway. We continued our vacation, with me spending a great deal of it in bed and my family members taking turns with me. My parents had arrived by this point, so the opposing team now included two more members. This rehab thing was going to happen.

I called Marilyn, my HPSP caseworker, to tell her what was going on. She said that because I hadn't yet started HPSP, that she wouldn't report me to the Board of Medical Practice, as long as I did not return to work but entered inpatient treatment as soon as the facility had an opening. I agreed. My parents changed their flights so that they could travel home with me and the kids. I remained sober, truthfully due to the "correctional officers" who were by my side the entire time, taking orders from my sister, the warden. I was indeed resentful towards her. She was messing up my entire life! Now, I couldn't return to work and had to go to rehab. How dare she try to keep me alive and my kids safe! Obviously, this is said with sarcasm and in hindsight, she was absolutely doing all of the right things. I was a complete mess, endangering myself, the kids, anyone on the road, my patients, and at risk of drinking myself to death. Yet at the time, I felt that they were unfairly ganging up on me.

I stayed sober for twelve days. Arriving home, my parents stayed with us. My father took care of the kids and my mother basically handcuffed herself to me. She took me to my first support group meeting. She took me to the chemical dependency evaluation that would seal my fate requiring inpatient treatment. My parents were so solid and unwavering. My mom even encouraged me to invite Michael over the night before admission so that I had someone to hold me during the night. So, he did. On the morning of admission, I snuck out of bed early, drove to Target to buy some yoga pants for rehab, and stopped at the liquor store the moment it opened. I drank a pint of vodka in the car before I even got home. I blew a .19 upon admission several hours later. I figured it was my last chance to drink so I took it. I was also so scared, and I knew that alcohol would calm me down. It did, temporarily.

Chapter Nine

DETOX #2

"You mean the twenty-eight days don't start until I am out of detox, and had I come in here sober I could have avoided detox?" I asked. Yes, that was the deal. If you come in loaded, they have to detox you first and however long you stay in detox does NOT count towards the twenty-eight days. So, I repeated the same Steps I had taken in detox #1. Slow exhale, special hand movements and tongue movements, the whole thing. I did not want to stay in detox any longer than I had to, because I still had almost a month to be locked up. I was not looking forward to it—at all. I did not think I really needed it and I was there to appease my family and keep my job and PA license. The wrong reasons for going to rehab are when you go for any other reason besides that you want to be sober. But, I was there. I was stuck, and there was nothing I could do about it. I got out of detox in forty-eight hours and was admitted to the professional women's floor at Hazelden, called Dia Linn.

REHAB #1

On my floor were other health care professionals, lawyers, accountants, and had there been any pilots or judges, they would have been there, too. It was a group of women that I could relate to, in terms of education level and career status. Many were married, many with kids. Some of these women had been here before, some even several times. Some had lost their careers, their homes, their marriages, their children, everything. I had not lost any of that, and I constantly compared myself to them, feeling much better about myself because I was not nearly as bad as they were. They kept telling me. "You haven't gotten the "yets" yet, Karla, but you will if you keep drinking" they would say. The "yets." I didn't believe this. I also believed I could stop drinking much easier than they did. I had a ton of willpower and determination; I should have no difficulty with rehab and sobriety.

I was introduced to the Twelve Steps. Classes in meditation, biofeedback, spirituality, relapse prevention, as well as daily process groups took place where you talk about your feelings. Ugh. I had always been an excellent student, and this was no different. I planned to ace these Steps and check them off my list, get out, and get on with my life. Jackie, my counselor, saw through my bullshit though. As I was working on emailing friends and family to apologize for my behavior (Step Nine), she asked me what step I was on. I told her, obviously, Step Nine. I had already completed the first Eight Steps. "No, Karla. You are on Step One." I did not agree. I was announcing myself as an alcoholic, I was in rehab; clearly I had accepted that I had a problem. I already believed in God, so Step Two and Step Three were crossed off. I had made my list of people I had harmed and knew the bad things I had done, and had told a lot of women in the group about those things, so Step Five—check. Six and seven were easy, only a couple of paragraphs in the Big Book, so they were complete. I had made my list of people I thought I had hurt (Step Eight), and was in a big hurry to gain their forgiveness and approval so I was on to Step Nine. She put a stop to that at once, even eliminating my email privileges.

Jackie wanted me to slow down. She tried to convince me that the Steps are not an assignment but a way of life, and that there is no rushing them. Also, you don't just complete the Steps one time and you graduate. It is a life-long commitment to working these Steps constantly in daily life. Well, that sounded ridiculous to me. I just wanted to get the Steps "done" and move on. I wanted to get back to normal, never mind that my normal had become completely screwed up and no one in their right mind would have desired my normal. But, I did. And I wanted it as soon as possible.

Trying to slow my pace, she assigned me to thirty minutes a day in the meditation room. No books, papers, nothing besides me in a quiet room. To a person like me at that time, with racing hamster wheel thoughts and severe anxiety and fear of the future, this was utter torture. I would look at the clock thinking I must be close to done, and only two minutes had passed!! She also had me complete many of my assignments with my non-dominant hand. Writing essays and lists with my left hand—all in an attempt to get me to slow down and accept imperfection. These exercises seemed stupid to me, but I had no choice but to keep on. I dug into my past, but truly only a little bit. I participated in groups, always saying or doing what I thought I should. I continued to keep up with the outside world, my parents and children coming twice a week for visiting hours, my mother sneaking in my phone so I could check emails and respond to texts. They brought in my bills so I could pay them. I refused any groups that were not mandatory, and spent a lot of time in my room. I read that Big Book of Alcoholics Anonymous from cover to cover—twice. But it didn't really sink in. The stories about other alcoholics in the second half of the book were about people who seemed so much worse than me, who had lost everything. That wasn't me. I did not feel I could relate, and once again, felt that I did not need to be there.

I became a mother figure to many in the group, listening to their problems, trying to offer sound advice, parroting sayings and things I had heard or read in treatment. I only disclosed my own personal stories when it was an assignment; otherwise I quickly turned conversations that involved vulnerability so that the spotlight was on someone else. I did not make any long lasting friends, because I did not want to. These were not my people. My counselor warned me about all of this, telling me I was a recipe for relapse if I didn't start to gain some acceptance of my own situation. I couldn't. I was not ready. Saying I was an alcoholic and believing it were two entirely different things. I certainly was not convinced that I had the disease of alcoholism. I checked boxes off the calendar counting down the days to my release. Hazelden tried to get me to stay longer, and attend an extended care program at the "Lodge," but this cost money out of pocket and required more time away from work and home and I refused. Jackie even went around me and asked my parents if they could help financially to keep me there longer. They wanted to, but I wouldn't let them, and I was furious that Jackie had gone to them. I felt that Hazelden was just a money-making machine and that they wanted to keep everyone there as long as possible to improve their bottom line. There may be some truth to that, but in hindsight, they knew what I needed. I have also since heard, countless times, that the "Lodge" is where many alcoholics truly found their way. I just couldn't or wouldn't see it at the time.

Finally, I was released. But that wasn't the end. They insisted on an aftercare program including something called Intensive Outpatient, or IOP. This would be five days a week for a month, and slowly drop from there depending on my progress. They were not allowing me to return to work, and if I did not adhere to their aftercare recommendations, they would report me to HPSP, who would then report me to the Board. I had no choice but to comply. My employer had been understanding and gracious, and I was on short-term disability so I was being paid enough to get by. My parents stayed with me for the first month following discharge. They had cared for my children during my inpatient stay, and somehow they had been able to keep it a secret from my ex-husband, Jim, so he couldn't use it against me and try to gain custody of the kids. My mother attended the Family Program at Hazelden and learned a great deal about enabling and boundaries. She learned about "detaching with love," which I certainly felt. My father and my sister, at the time, were not interested, and had simply detached. They were angry, rightly so. My sister was still not taking my calls.

Mom and Dad returned to their home, and I continued to take my kids to school, go to IOP, and pick them up after. There were urine screens occasionally at IOP. These people were like me in that they were all forced to be there, but unlike me, most of them were young punks in all sorts of trouble; some even on jail release to attend. I had thought I had nothing in common with the residential treatment groups but in IOP, I really felt out of place. I figured out how the system worked, I realized what I had to do to satisfy the requirements, but the anxiety and fear and racing thoughts did not abate. In fact, they became stronger. I was resentful of being stuck in the rooms at IOP. I was resentful that I hadn't been allowed to return to work. I was never grateful for sobriety or that I still had my job, or kids, or home. I did not even attempt to learn real tools to use to help me figure out why it was that I drank, so that I could not drink again. I was white knuckling it again and resentments, angers, and fears were building by the minute. It is said that resentments are poison for an alcoholic. It is the truth.

I remained sober about two weeks into IOP, so a total of about six weeks including inpatient rehab. I stored a whole bunch of my clean urine in tiny washed out five-hour energy bottles in the freezer. I learned about this on the internet—"how to fake a urine drug test." Every day, I would thaw out a little bottle, for they contained just over 30 ml of urine, which was enough for a sample. I would heat it in hot water until a thermometer read 98 degrees or so, and I would place that little bottle intravaginally so it would stay at body temperature (because they test for temp as well as drugs and alcohol), and that way I had it with me in the event they asked for a sample. I allowed myself to start drinking. Again, first at night only. Then, right after class. Then, before class as well. I chewed gum. I was never asked for a breath test or another urine test during the remainder of my time in IOP. Nobody ever knew. Upon graduation, my counselor said such kind things about me. None of those things were true. But, I had gotten by with it.

During IOP, I met a man, Mark, who was several years younger than me. While I was an inpatient, my counselor Jackie had convinced me to break things off with Michael once and for all. I had done that. But, I was lonely and craving love. I hated myself, so I had to find love from other people, and I had managed to alienate so many of my friends and family members. It was pounded into all of us at rehab that dating or embarking upon new romantic relationships within the first year of sobriety are a terrible idea. Well, I wasn't sober anymore, so that didn't seem pertinent. Mark was a cocaine addict. Tall, mean eyes, big and angry—a take control type of man. Just the type I seem to be attracted to. He had never been married nor did he have children, he said his drinking and drugging always ruined relationships. Nonetheless, I forged ahead and embarked upon an intense relationship with him, full of extreme highs and lows, with both of our addictions running the show. He would disappear for days on a cocaine bender. He would show up at my house and we would fight, and then make up. The kids liked him, even my ex-husband seemed to like him. Mark was a gentle giant, a kind and sweet man when sober. Mean, abusive and paranoid when high on coke. He blamed our problems on my drinking; I blamed our problems on his cocaine.

Having graduated from IOP, I was subsequently required to step down to a less time consuming treatment, three mornings a week. The Haven, a center in Woodbury, MN, took me on. It was a small group, it was fine. But of course, I was drinking daily by this time. My life consisted of a totally dysfunctional relationship, daily drinking, attending treatment three days a week, bringing my little bottles of clean urine wherever I went in case I had to do a UA. At the request of my children, I put a voluntary ignition interlock system in my car. They were familiar with these devices, because their dad had been required to get one following his DWI. I set it up for the minimum; the car would start if I blew anything under .08. If I blew over that, it wasn't reported anywhere, the car simply wouldn't start. This provided some security to the kids that at least I couldn't drive them around over the legal limit. The system required a start blow, another one in five minutes, and then every twenty minutes following. Any time I shut off the engine, the process started over again if I were to attempt to restart. About this time, I was allowed to return to work on a part time basis. Hallelujah!

Once returning to work, I had to begin calling in to the HPSP color line every morning and provide a urine sample if my color was called. The clinic for which I worked was an authorized collection site. Although I didn't want to break my anonymity, it was the most convenient place to provide samples, as the sample had to be collected by 6 pm. I went the first time, with my little bottle of urine tucked inside me, gave the sample, and Emily, a friend and patient of mine who ran the lab, told me I could come in the back way anytime I needed this done. She would be there for me and keep it private, no checking in and no sitting in the waiting room. She was so kind. And I totally took advantage of her kindness. I figured out how to bypass any collection site and just forge Emily's signature and send in the kits myself to HPSP. This meant if my color was called, I could just pop a sample out of the freezer and throw it in the collection kit without the whole mess of thawing out, carrying it around, and bothering Emily. It was so easy.

However, I was going to run out of urine and knew that I couldn't use my own. My eight-year-old daughter had frequent UTI's, so she was used to providing samples so I could check for UTI's at home. I began asking her to pee in a bucket often so I could "check it," and then saving HER urine in those little bottles for future use. The system was working perfectly. I was able to work, be a mom, have my relationship and drink. I forged signatures from Mary, a woman I had seen at a meeting, and called her my sponsor on paper. I had never even talked to her, just heard her say her name. I did not yet need a counselor or doctor as I was still attending outpatient, which satisfied HPSP. I was totally faking the whole deal. I was getting by with it, and that boosted my ego and made me feel so smart. The house of cards would not stand much longer.

I found out that my ex, Jim, was going to have a baby with his new girlfriend. This crushed me. He had never wanted another baby with me, but now he was having one with her. Why hadn't I been good enough? The self-pity was enormous and the hit to my self-esteem dramatic. I felt such emotional and even physical pain with this revelation. I felt an out of proportion amount of sadness, considering it had been my choice to divorce him. Yet, it really, really hurt. I would lie there at night, with my headphones playing sad Vince Gill and Amy Winehouse songs, pining over what could have been—what I threw away. I was missing a toxic relationship. My mind was a total mess.

Little did I know, at the time that I was also pregnant. Mark and I were very excited, as were the kids. My family was supportive; they thought that a pregnancy would mean I would be determined to stay sober. I wanted to. I wanted the baby so badly and of course wanted it to be healthy. But I simply could not stop drinking. The deals I made in my own brain about drinking were insane. I read that alcohol does not really affect a fetus until the end of the first trimester which eased my mind, but then I would read another article that reported effects of alcohol on the fetus were from the moment of conception. I was terrified that I was hurting my baby; I know the effects of fetal alcohol syndrome, the risks of alcoholic mothers and childbirth, the high risk of miscarriage and a multitude of other serious complications due to active alcoholism. I would try in the mornings not to take that first drink. Shaking, vomiting, nauseated, anxious, I couldn't resist the "cure." My body and my brain were screaming for the drink. I rationalized and thought if I slowly cut down I would be done drinking by the time that second trimester arrived. I continued to work and attempted to be a good mother, but alcohol remained my number one priority. I could not understand how I had been able to stop with my other pregnancies but could not this time. It was a war within myself that was so destructive and painful it is almost impossible to describe. I would pray, and ask God for help, but secretly felt that I didn't deserve God's help or mercy. I would sob and I hated myself. The guilt and shame and hopelessness of the situation were overwhelming.

In short order, Mark moved in with me and the kids. Blissful cohabitation was not to be, however. He would go missing for a day or two, and return apologetic and full of guilt because he had been using cocaine again. He would sleep it off for a couple of days. Meanwhile, I was drinking and he would find me passed out on the floor with the kids fending for themselves and verbalize that my drinking was not good for the baby or for his recovery. I knew that, but I still couldn't stop. We used each other as scapegoats and accused and shamed each other, so that we would have one fewer reason to point the finger at ourselves. One day, he came home high. I was cooking something that contained red meat, which he avoided due to his feelings that the treatment of animals for human consumption was horrid. We fought—about MEAT. The fight escalated until, to my recollection, he threw a bowl of macaroni and cheese at me (for some reason, it seems men like to throw food at me). He started throwing things around the room. I told him to get out of my house. He told me that it was his house now, too, and he was not leaving. I threatened to call the police. He got angrier. I threatened to call his father, and he lost it. He slapped me twice across the face, told me I was a worthless drunk, told me that he was smarter than me, and told me he could kill me right then if he wanted to. He took a pillow and threatened to smother me with it. The kids were witnessing this entire nightmare, and the three of us somehow got into my son's bedroom and locked the door.

We could hear him smashing things, yelling, shouting curse words. I called the police, who ultimately arrested him for assault and terroristic threats. When told that the argument began due to a disagreement about red meat, one of the police officers said "I've heard worse." Really? A knock down drag out over meat? The final straw was that when they were about to take Mark away to the police station, I told them I thought Mark had taken my purse and keys. They found them in the trunk of his car, which solidified their case against him. He spent a couple days in jail. I got a restraining order against him and hired movers the next day to remove all of his things to a storage unit. I recall sitting in my truck with the kids, drinking vodka, watching the movers haul things into the storage unit, wondering how I had gotten here, knowing that the bottle in my hand was destroying my life, and the lives of those around me, including my tiny baby. The pregnancy did not survive. Ultimately, I dropped the charges against Mark. He went on with his life, and me with mine. Broken.

My parents arrived quickly to help pick up the pieces, literally and figuratively. They swept up broken glass, held and hugged me, tried to discuss my drinking. Feeling so hopeless and like such a complete and utter failure, my drinking picked up even more, although I realize that doesn't seem possible. I felt sadness and emptiness, guilt and shame. I had wanted another child so badly, yet here I was. I tried to fill that hole with booze. And more booze. And even more booze. My mother found every last bottle and dumped them down the drain. I resorted to cooking sherry—which is terrible, but did the job. My father disabled my car so that I couldn't drive, my mother took my purse. I still was able, when they were away from the house, to steal cash from my ten year old and borrow a car to drive to a liquor store and buy more. My mother found this stash and dumped it as well. I begged and pleaded and told her I couldn't safely just stop, I had to be in detox or tapered from the alcohol. She then, begrudgingly, went to buy more vodka for me. She gave me a shot every hour or so, with the intention to taper. I tore the house up looking for that bottle. My mother was a better hide and seek player than I was. I never did find it.

We decided—well they decided and I just hazily agreed that it would be best if I took the kids and moved in with my parents. I quit my job, with no notice. We packed up a bunch of clothes and other necessities. We packed up the cats and their food and litter. A caravan was formed of my dad in the lead in his car, followed by drunken me and the cats, followed still by my mother carrying my babies. We stopped once in a while so that my mom could distribute a shot of alcohol to me. The kids were enrolled in a new school as the new school year was about to begin. My mother continued to detox me slowly at home, and it actually began to work.

In all of this chaos, I had not been calling in regularly to my monitoring agency and missed a screen. My caseworker notified me of this. Although I was currently between jobs, I was hoping to get a PA position in my parents' community. I did not want to lose my license. My caseworker told me that if I didn't want the board involved, I needed to go to a local collection site and leave an observed sample. OBSERVED!! How in the world was I going to pass an observed test? My drinking had certainly decreased with the help "my mother's treatment center," but I would still never pass a test. Terrified, I began researching ways to pass an observed drug test online, and it was shocking all of the suggestions I found. Within the supplies I had packed, I had brought a small cooler of ice with several of those tiny bottles of my daughter's frozen urine. But, an observed test meant they were going to watch me urinate. I learned a technique online and practiced over and over. Using one of those five-hour energy bottles, removing the cover and replaced it with a layer of tinfoil secured with a rubber band. This was placed tinfoil side down inside my vagina. Then, when it was time to hold the cup under my urine stream, I punctured the tinfoil with my pinky fingernail, and voila. I was so nervous. Nervous the bottle would leak or rupture accidentally. Nervous that the collection site would use a toilet hat instead of a cup which would remove my ability to puncture the tinfoil. The lengths I was going to keep drinking were astounding. It worked. I passed the test—by cheating. What had I become? I vowed that if I passed that test, this would be it. I would not drink again. Another broken promise to myself.

With my wits more about me, I began to search for jobs and actually was offered a position. Before I could accept, however, my ex-husband Jim got involved. Since we shared legal custody of the children, I could not legally transfer them to a different school without his agreement. He did not agree. I talked with my attorney, with my family; we tried to come up with a plan that would work. We could not. As quickly as our whirlwind move up north had happened, just as quickly the entire situation was reversed. But now, I had a few days sobriety. I felt like I could do this. Tearfully, my mother bid us farewell and off we went, the kids, the cats, our belongings, back home. I made it as far as the liquor store nearest home before stopping to buy a bottle which I started drinking in the car because I couldn't wait the two miles until we got home.

I called my previous employer, begging for my position back. They were wary and insisted on a meeting with the higher ups of the organization. At the meeting, we discussed my prior treatment, my leave of absence, my worsening attendance record as I had begun calling in sick once or twice a month. I pleaded my case. They listened. They took some time to deliberate, and ultimately decided that I was too risky of a provider to hire back. I was devastated. I even went so far as to call the chair of the family practice department, drunk, and begged him for my job. Needless to say, it was not successful.

Because of the circumstances in which I had left my job, with the restraining order and police report, I was able to qualify for unemployment benefits. I continued to pay cobra for health insurance. I had a couple hundred thousand dollars in 401K's that I knew I could tap into if needed. I deferred my mortgage. I tried to find another position, but that was taking a lot of time. I got the kids to and from school, drank all day, and became more depressed and lonely than I thought possible. My mother checked in on me often over the phone, my friends Maureen, Patty, and Jeanne tried to reach out. I rarely answered the phone. I didn't answer the door. I began to call in sick for the kids to school often so that I didn't have to worry about driving them there and back. If I did drive them, I recall wondering if any of the other moms in the drop off or pick up line were drunk and horrible like me. I was becoming more confused and paranoid, not always knowing what day it was, or if I awoke and the clock said 5:00, I had no idea if it was A.M. or P.M. At the last minute I remembered that it was school conference time for my son. I flew out of bed (it was the middle of the afternoon), wearing a tattered sweater, capri cargo pants, long wool socks, and flip-flops, with my hair matted, drunk and my skin pasty. This is how I arrived to meet the 5th grade teacher that day.

On another afternoon, I had scheduled the kids to attend an after school program but forgot. I arrived to meet the school bus after school and found my kids not on it. I panicked. I chased down the school bus. I got it to pull over as I feverishly tried to get them to understand that my kids were supposed to be on that bus. After speeding to school to look for them there, I found them quietly playing in the Adventure Club room, just like they were supposed to be. Just like I had arranged but forgotten. Another particularly bad day, I even called the national suicide hotline while in the line to pick up the kids and hung up when the kids got in the car. I was spiraling fast and taking the kids down with me, and had no earthly idea how to stop the progression.

Besides the guardian ad litem I had hired to "protect the kids from Jim," I also had them enrolled in therapy for a couple of years with an awesome counselor named Jonathan. He saw them a couple of times a month. In my paranoid state, I thought that if I didn't show up with the kids to therapy, Jonathan would wonder what was going on and find me out. I drove the kids to therapy, drunk. I had a new 1.75 of brandy in the passenger seat. I nearly hit a light pole when we parked. I told the kids, ages eight and ten, to go in by themselves and check in and come out when they were done with their session. I drank and passed out in the car.

My children, who had become more adult-like than I was, told on me to Jonathan. He came out to the car and banged on the passenger window until I came to. He was kind, but firm, took the bottle, and told me to come inside with him. He called Jim. He called the guardian ad litem, Matthew. I sat in the waiting room crying and scared while these three men decided my fate. They came to the gracious decision that if I was able to find a sober person to come get me, leave my car there, and drive me directly to detox, they would not get the police involved. This was a gift. At the time, I did not even realize what a gift, as I would have been facing DWI, open container, child endangerment, and probably many other charges.

I was able to find someone from my prior outpatient treatment (remember the "young punks" I referred to previously), a young man named Cal who was sober and local and came straight away. We had not spoken since graduation months previously, and I still don't know exactly why he agreed to help me, but he did. He took me home to pack a few things. Jim, with the children, followed to pick up a supply of clothing and necessities for the kids. They were now going to live with him, indefinitely, while I tried to get my shit together.

Chapter Ten

DETOX #3

Back to Fairview Riverside I went, first through the ER. I was a piece of shit and the ER staff knew it. They began the whole ordeal again—labs, Ativan, IV fluids with multivitamins. My liver enzymes were through the roof. I was malnourished and dehydrated. I had head lice. I had lost so much weight that I was just a pale bag of bones. Once I was stable, up to the detox floor I went.

This time, I did not refuse the Ativan. I did not fake any of the tests that were administered to assess withdrawal symptoms. I attended groups and meetings, and I truly wanted to get sober. I was going to lose my children completely if I didn't get this figured out. They offered a twenty-one day treatment to me upon detox discharge, but did not have any openings right away. They told me that they would have an opening within a few days, but I had to stay sober in order to enroll. They would not take me into treatment drunk and I would have to go through detox again and be put on the waiting list again.

I went home, took a cab to get there because I was too broken and ashamed to ask anyone for help. I managed, miracle of miracles, to stay sober those three days. I informed my monitoring agency of the situation and they "fired" me from their program and reported me to the Board of Medical Practice. I talked with the guardian ad litem, who assured me that if I successfully completed treatment, I would be able to see my children, albeit with a paid supervisor at first. I was filled with unimaginable fear. But the fear of never seeing my children again kept me sober those three days. I called the treatment center every hour on the hour, as they had encouraged me to do, to check if they had any open treatment beds. Finally, they did. Again, not wanting to ask for help, I packed up for a twenty-one day stay, and drove my own car to the parking ramp attached to the hospital, paid for a monthly pass, and was directly admitted.

ᴄᴧᴏChapter Eleven ᴄᴧᴏ

REHAB #2

This was not at all as severely restricted as the detox floor. We were not to bring our phones, though I did and assumed they would put it in lockdown upon arrival. They did not. There were no clothing or makeup restrictions. You could go downstairs to eat at the Subway restaurant within the hospital if you had a break and money, wander to the pharmacy to pick up some candy or whatever you wanted, walked to and from larger meeting rooms scattered throughout the hospital, and basically were free except during the mandatory classes.

This is not to say that the days were unstructured, they were not. There was just a lot more freedom and breaks than what I had experienced at detox, or at Hazelden a few months previously. I was required to take a urine drug screen upon arrival as well as perform a breath test, both of which I passed, without faking this time! I was assigned a roommate, whose name sadly escapes me. She was an opiate addict, and was attempting a suboxone treatment plan in which they were constantly titrating and changing her medication regimen. This rendered her often sleeping and near comatose. I basically had the room to myself. After the evening meal and mandatory seven p.m. speaker meeting, I retired to my room for the remainder of the evening to read and enjoy the blissful solitude in which I had begun to find such comfort because of my drinking.

Something was missing, however. It was social interaction, connectedness, feeling that I belonged. I did not have that, nor was I about to entertain that. Making long lasting friendships was not part of my plan. I just wanted to get my twenty-one days completed, and get back to my life and my kids, in whatever capacity that would mean to the guardian ad litem. Totally off script, I actually met someone there, a lovely woman named Lauren, whom I briefly referred to in the very first chapter of this book. She was a few years older than me, with nineteen-year-old triplet girls. Her girls were not speaking to her. She was an alcoholic like me, with four DWI's under her belt. She was there out of necessity. She had recently been diagnosed with a very aggressive and deadly type of breast cancer. Her oncologist would not begin chemo or radiation treatments until she got sober. She was funny as hell, kind, real and raw, and I don't believe I have ever felt such an instant connection with another woman, and we became friends rapidly. She is still one of my best friends and favorite people on the planet.

But even with this newfound friendship, I still felt lacking and uncomfortable. I was participating in the groups, but nothing was sinking in. I was hearing tragic stories of loss and tribulations related to alcoholism, but it did not seem to motivate me. I began to notice the freedoms we had more acutely. I realized that they were not asking for random UA's or breath tests on anyone. I had a special allowance to go to the parking garage every couple of days and start my car, as it was winter in Minnesota, and I was fearful it wouldn't start when it was time to leave. Although I didn't dare risk driving away from the ramp and trying to come back, I did gain confidence in that nobody seemed to notice or care regarding my absence on these car starting jaunts. About a week into my treatment, I took a chance. I tucked my hospital nametag in my shirt, grabbed my purse and keys, started the car and stopped it again, and left the ramp through the side door on foot where I hailed a cab. Asking the driver to take me to the nearest liquor store resulted in a funny look. I made up some story about how my sister had just had a baby, and we were Russian and needed vodka to celebrate. Turns out, the funny look was not because he cared WHY I wanted to go to the liquor store. The real reason for his confusion became apparent very quickly when after approximately a one block drive, we arrived at the liquor store. He asked if he should wait to drive me back, I sheepishly told him I thought I could manage the block by foot. I bought two 1.75 liters of cheap vodka and walked back to the parking garage. I put the booze in the car, but not before taking a couple of swigs.

75

Giant sigh of relief. It was like magic. This is what I had been missing. This would fill the gaping hole in my being. Upon filling my water bottle with the glorious liquid, I put my nametag back on and left the parking ramp to join my next group.

Though never getting drunk or obvious, I sipped vodka out of my water bottle throughout the remainder of my treatment. My roommate never noticed; of course she was sleeping most of the time. No one in any of the groups said anything; the counselor and addiction doctor seemed to think things were going well for me. My friend, Lauren, told me she never had a clue. My nighttime retreats to read in bed now were so much better because I could drink—though I think I read the same section of my book every night, not recalling what I had read the night before. As an aside, two days prior to discharge, I got a new roommate. She was an alcoholic. She swore she was losing her mind because she felt like she smelled vodka in our room. Imagine that!

The guardian ad litem, Matthew, came to visit me at treatment shortly before discharge. He met with me and my counselor, and I received a stellar report card. Matthew discussed that I should look into paid parenting time supervisors, because that would be the first step in seeing my kids. I was going to have to pay someone to babysit me while I spent time with my children. My own children! I was willing to do anything, except quit drinking to do so, so I said I would do it. I still had the financial reserves to afford this, despite being on unemployment without any foreseeable employment opportunities. I hired a woman that Matthew recommended named Tammy. She would come the next week on a Saturday afternoon for four hours. Jim would bring the kids to me at the same time. Although this wasn't at all what I was hoping for, it was a start.

On the day of discharge, I said my goodbyes, got my graduation chip (in recovery, milestones are often celebrated with small chips or key chains or other tokens to commemorate the amount of time one has been sober), and took my bags to the car. I had forgotten, however, about the ignition interlock. Damn! I was too drunk to start my own car right after leaving a twenty-one day treatment program. Who does that? So, I walked around the parking ramp in the cold to try to burn off the alcohol. It took 2 ½ hours before I could blow below a .08 and start the car. Then, after driving, I blew at the five-minute mark, and knew I would make it home before I had to blow again. So, I began drinking in the car. The very next day, I had the ignition interlock removed from my car. In my alcoholic mind, it was simply too much of a hassle.

Attempting to plan for the future, and now having the Board of Medical Practice involved, I was not going to be able to get a PA job while my license was under investigation. I would qualify for another five months of unemployment, but had to plan for beyond that. Wanting to continue to drink, and exhausted from the restrictions and monitoring that HPSP came with, I honestly considered hanging up my stethoscope. I researched opening up a home daycare and becoming licensed. Because who doesn't want a drunk daycare provider! First things first, though, I was going to get to see my kids.

The parenting time supervisor, Tammy, was set to arrive at the house at 4 pm. Jim was going to bring the kids about that same time. He arrived before she did, and I convinced him to go ahead and leave them there. I had a few minutes alone with them before she arrived. I hugged them, I cried, I promised them that I was better and that I would be better. I ran to the closet every chance I got to drink. The pressure was getting to me. Tammy arrived. I played "Candyland" with the kids escaping to the bedroom closet between turns for a swig of vodka. Then I made them some dinner. I remember feeling inexplicably sad and hopeless; trying to simply make dinner for my own children was such a challenge. She was watching me—what if she didn't think what I fed them was nutritious? What if she thought I was a bad Mom? What if I didn't do well and she told the guardian? I kept sneaking off to make take a drink. The kids and Tammy sat down at the table to eat. I excused myself, and ended up in the coat closet with my bottle, sobbing, which is where Tammy found me. She was kind, she rubbed my back and told me it would be OK, but the visit was officially over, and she reported to the guardian that I was unfit to be unsupervised with the children and that until I got real help; she was no longer willing to be my supervisor.

There was no promise of seeing my kids in the near future, or ever for that matter, no job or career, no family, no relationship, nothing. Even my lawyer had fired me. I was emotionally, spiritually and physically bankrupt and I had allowed alcohol to steal everything from me. I spiraled even faster than ever before. My life revolved around drinking and sleeping. I didn't shower or eat. I crawled around the house trying to find a place comfortable enough to sleep. I got to the point where I was unable to actually walk down a flight of stairs, I was too weak. I had to sit down and slowly scoot, one step at a time, like a toddler. All I could keep down was vodka and PowerAde—and neither of those options was even a given. There was so much vomiting and heaving. There was crying. I went so far as to reach out to Michael, the married surgeon I had previously been involved with. I asked him to come and give me some IV fluids at my home, because I was really sick but I did not want to go back to detox or treatment. He did. But, after 2 liters, I still didn't feel much better and he was not comfortable giving any more. I asked him to leave, I wanted to be alone. At some point during these couple of days, I have cloudy recollections of my friends Jeanne, Maureen, and Patty checking on me. I refused everyone's attempt to take me to the hospital. I sent them all away. I was probably as close to death as humans can get without actually dying. I wanted to die. The pain was too great. I was filthy, both outside and inside. I could not see the point of going on in this life. I felt that the lives of my children and family, and society in general, would be much better if

I were not around. I truly believed this. I was a horrible person. I had done unspeakable things. I had thrown away a life that many people can't even dream of having. There seemed absolutely no hope.

I dragged a giant basket of leftover medications, vitamins and pills of all sorts, into my closet with my liquor, my laptop, and my phone. And then, a real miracle happened.

I called Phil.

The rehab broker on the pop up that appeared on my computer while researching suicide.

And together, we began to save my life.

Chapter Twelve

DETOX #4

The IV fluids must have made some difference after all, for me to have functioned well enough to get on that plane and get to Orlando. After drinking my last two tiny bottles of vodka in the toilet stall of the Orlando International Airport, I went to meet my transport to "The Recovery Village" in Umatilla, Florida—the middle of nowhere. There was a young woman, Jess, from Missouri also going to the same center. We were transported in the same van and subsequently put together as roommates. She was a meth and opiate addict. She had been in the same public restroom as me at the airport, snorting her last two Percocet tablets in another toilet stall. She was young, only in her early twenties. I was old enough to be her mother, but we got along great from the first "hello."

It was after midnight, early Thanksgiving Day 2013, when Jess and I were admitted to rehab. This was different. The staff was kind and understanding, but also all-knowing with an uncanny ability to call bullshit when it was warranted. They did not seem to look at me as a piece of garbage, but as a human being. Or, perhaps, since this whole rehab try had actually been my idea, instead of being pushed into it from one outside force or another, I was just ready. Finally ready to end the nightmare that had become my life.

We were checked in, our purses and phones were taken, our belongings were thoroughly examined, and we were taken to our room. Three queen beds with fluffy white down comforters, polished hardwood floors, a regular bathroom with a real door, and a flat screen TV were in our room. We were each assigned a bed, mine in the middle, Jess' nearest the door, and the one by the window remained empty throughout our stay. The detox nurse, knowing that I was coming in drunk and would be facing withdrawal soon, spent a great deal of time with me. He wanted to know how my previous detox's had gone. He explained to me the importance of taking the Ativan he would be offering, as it would help to clear my system and actually get my head clear enough to attend groups much sooner than if I tried to fight it. I was ready to listen. I took his advice. In fact, from that moment on, I took all the advice any of the staff gave me and followed recommendations precisely. I was ready for help and I was ready to take that help without trying to control the situation or get in my own way.

Detox was actually not bad. I was given the Ativan every four hours or so, slowly tapering down the dosage and frequency over three days until I no longer needed it. I was given a medication called Gabapentin, which helps with seizure risk as well as a host of other recovery related things. I saw the addiction medicine specialist, who prescribed Lexapro for my generalized anxiety, and trazodone, a non-addictive sleep aid. In the past, I had refused these medications. Sometimes it was out of pride (I don't need that, that won't work for me, I am not like "those" people who can't deal with their anxiety or depression), and sometimes it was because I had tried it and it hadn't helped me in the past— trazodone in particular. Of course, when I had tried it, I had also been drinking myself into oblivion every night. I wouldn't have been able to tell if it helped or not! My goal had been to pass out, not gently fall asleep.

The medications began to really make a difference. The fog cleared, but this time, probably because of the meds and because I was truly ready, I did not get the uncomfortable, irritable, restless feelings and cravings for the drink that I had previously had following detox. I slowly became part of the living, and was discharged from detox to the main rehabilitation program. Jess detoxed at about the same speed.

Chapter Thirteen

REHAB #3

The facility was nearly at capacity, so there was no room for us to physically move to the general floor, and Jess and I were housed on the detox floor for nearly a whole month. This was a nice perk, because the general floor did not have TV's in the rooms but the detox rooms did. The general floor did not have 24/7 snacks available, but the detox area did. And, the detox floor was quiet and removed from the chaos of the general floor, which I liked very much. We were eventually moved to the general floor, where Jess and I continued to be roommates, for nearly the entirety of my sixty-four day stay.

The facility had three outdoor courtyards. One was for smokers, which I had never been but became while I was there. The second, outside the detox area, was tranquil and lush. And the third, a charming area with umbrella covered tables and chairs and chaise lounges, was complete with a koi pond. Out another door there was a pool, basketball court, and picnic tables. It felt very relaxing and lovely to me and so much better than the previous centers I had attended. Looking back, Hazelden had been very posh, having a much better reputation among rehab centers, with even more amenities. But, I had felt like it was jail because I wasn't ready and did not want to be there, and I definitely didn't want to be sober. This time was different. I had nothing left to lose because I had already lost it. I was there for me. *To save my own life.* Not to please anyone else. I did not know if I would ever see my children again, even if I was able to get sober. I did not have a job to go back to, and didn't even know if I would ever be allowed to practice medicine again. I had (correction: my mother had) put my home on the market prior to leaving. There was no way I could continue to keep that big house from a financial standpoint. So, I may not even have a home to go "home" to. My sister wasn't taking my calls, nor was my father or many of my friends, so I did not know if I would ever have a normal relationship with them in the future. I was doing this for me, and if successful, knew that I would be truly starting my life over again. That was daunting, but I was at peace.

"Sam has been assigned to be your counselor," the tech told me. I didn't know any of the counselors so that sounded fine to me. As the tech walked away, another patient said "You are SO lucky! He is amazing! I wish he was my counselor." Others echoed this sentiment. I couldn't wait to meet this man with such a reputation. I didn't need to wait long, for he came to find me shortly thereafter. Sam was maybe fifteen or twenty years older than me. Average height and build, with shoulder length flowing greyish brown hair and a matching mustache, he was dressed casually. He was not imposing, he was not frightening. My other counselors had all seemed scary to me, possibly because I felt that they held my livelihood (notice I did not say "life") in their hands. With Sam, though, he held my life. I felt an immediate connection with him. He had over twenty-five years sobriety under his belt and had been doing this for a long time. He knew his stuff, talked the talk, but also walked the walk. He knew lies and manipulation when he saw them, he knew truth, he knew addiction and the destruction that accompanies it, and potential pitfalls within sobriety. He had so much personal and career experience that there was no problem, issue, sin, or fear that I could bring up that surprised him.

He asked me to tell him my story—my history. After several sessions of me talking about my childhood, college, marriage, drinking, my life story, he had a fantastic grasp of who I was and how and why I had ended up there. It was time to start taking the Steps, for real this time. Not to check boxes off a list, but to truly work them. Thus began some of the hardest work of my life.

Step One

"We admitted we were powerless over alcohol— that our lives had become unmanageable"

This is, undoubtedly, the most important Step. I had to absolutely face the fact that my life had been completely destroyed, and there were two reasons for it: me, and alcohol. I was no longer drinking, I was clear headed, but I would most certainly return to my crutch of alcohol if I didn't "fix" me. My crutch had worked for a very long time. But, like crutches for a broken leg, you can't continue to use the crutches forever after your injury, you have to learn to get by without them in order to truly heal, recover, and get on with life. It's no different with alcohol. I had to admit that I was, without a doubt, an alcoholic, and that it had ruined my life and tried to kill me. I needed to figure out why I had nearly let it do so. I had to understand why I had come to rely on it, face my past and my fears and my flaws head-on or this addiction was going to win and take my life.

The 12 Steps, from my experience, need to be taken in order at first. There is a reason for the way it is set up. I have heard it compared to mathematics. It would be ridiculous to attempt to master calculus if you had not learned to add or subtract. Same with these Steps—to attempt to jump to Step Nine (apologizing to those I had hurt) without first firmly admitting I was an alcoholic and could not manage my own life would be a recipe for disaster. I had tried that at Hazelden to just get them done and make everyone forgive and love me as soon as possible. It does not work that way. It certainly didn't work for me.

I also learned that there is no timeline or completion, a very difficult thing to grasp for someone who had always been task and goal oriented. I will never finish working the Steps. It's a continuum of working them daily, a way of life. Now, with over five years of sobriety, I am working several Steps simultaneously and daily. Like a diabetic who can control and manage his diabetes with diet, exercise, medications, and insulin but is never "cured," the same can be said about alcoholism. I will never be cured. But the Steps help me manage it and prevent it from killing me.

Back to Step One—was I an alcoholic? I think that this is well documented in all of the chapters leading up to this one. It's odd, though, that my mind still wanted to challenge this. Alcoholism nagged at me and tried to convince me that I didn't really have a problem. Walter Anderson once wrote "Our lives only improve when we are willing to take chances and the first and most difficult risk we can take is to be honest with ourselves." True, yet so very difficult.

To help in admitting I was an alcoholic and that my life had become unmanageable, Sam asked me to write a list of what happens to me when I drink. As with many tasks, I took this one on to the point of near exhaustion. Here is the first part of my list, in no particular order of importance:

1.   Make bad choices
2.   Stop eating

3. Vomit
4. Experience insomnia
5. Drive drunk
6. Lose job
7. Lose financial stability
8. Lose kids
9. Miss work
10. Isolate
11. Let down those who love me
12. Neglect my kids
13. Risk my kids' safety
14. Risk my safety
15. Risk the safety of the general public
16. Cry
17. Become depressed
18. Experience debilitating anxiety
19. Become angry
20. Become suicidal
21. Become mean to loved ones
22. Become physically weak
23. Damage my liver
24. Become anemic
25. Bruise easily
26. Scare loved ones
27. Drunk dial
28. Lose weight
29. Partake in risky sex
30. Lie
31. Steal

32. Cheat
33. Manipulate
34. Compromise my morals
35. Experience headaches
36. Experience shakes
37. Stop basic hygiene
38. Lose my independence
39. Stop exercising
40. Stop caring about important events like birthdays and holidays
41. Lose the trust of my kids and other loved ones
42. Feel despair
43. Feel hopelessness
44. Feel a failure
45. Stop playing piano
46. Lose touch with God
47. Experience poor memory
48. Experience blackouts
49. Waste time that I can never get back
50. Become unreliable, unemployable, not dependable, unfit mother....

This list goes on and on but the point is, I did terrible things and became a person I didn't recognize or even like when I drank. In fact, I hated myself. It was becoming pretty clear that I was an alcoholic and could finally admit it. To take this one step further, Sam suggested that I write a goodbye letter to alcohol. He recommended I think about it as a relationship.

My dearest alcohol,

There is no easy way to say or do this and I am certain this is much harder on me than it is on you, but I cannot continue this relationship any longer. Things were seemingly so amazing between us for so long and I hold dearly many memories with you that are good. Parties, dancing, intimacy, laughter, holidays, travel, college, weddings, and so much more seemed better with you in my life. But then, I crossed the line. I began to abuse you. Then, I became obsessed with you. A very unhealthy obsession. You were my everything. I couldn't and wouldn't do anything without you. Instead of enhancing my life, our relationship became sick and so one-sided. I started to lose myself in you. I stopped caring about how I looked. I stopped eating. I became isolated from friends and family. I slept with you. I would vomit and shake if I didn't have you. A great majority of my life was spent tracking you down, bringing you home, spending as much time with you as possible. My family and friends began to despise you for taking me away from them. Instead of letting you go, I clung tighter. But, I had to go to great lengths to try to keep you a secret from everyone else. I chose you over my children, my friends, my family. I thought they were wrong for hating you. I didn't think our relationship was a problem—I still thought you were the only thing keeping me sane. The truth is, it was insane to continue on with you. I jeopardized everything that had been important to me. I compromised my morals, alienated loved ones, and became depressed, anxious and suicidal. My health failed.

Attempting "breaks" from you never lasted very long and I would come running back to you with determination to keep the relationship "normal." Yet each time only proved a worse obsession and further abuse. I became a different person. I often didn't work, pick up the phone, or take the time to bathe because I wanted to be with you. You were my life. My only friend. My lover. You let me down so many times, but I let myself down much worse. I knew how terrible I felt after one of our nights together, filled with crying and anger and turmoil. Yet, I kept coming back to you. I even stopped praying except an occasional prayer that God would just let me die because my pain and losses were so great. I still didn't want to face the fact that our relationship was the source of my problems. I was in denial. I loved you and only you. I was so selfish. You have hurt me, but not beyond repair. I am ending this relationship now. I fear you now. We can't have a casual relationship or see each other occasionally. I am fully aware that being with you even for a minute would lead to disaster beyond what we've already been through. It has to be a clean break. I know I will think of you often at first, and remember both good and bad times. I may see you in a store, or when I go out to eat, or even on TV. But be warned—I will not associate with you ever again. If we meet at a party or event, I may glance your way but I will not embrace you or touch you, though I may be tempted. I will remember the horrible times and what I lost and could lose by picking up where we left off. I have renewed my trust and reliance on God, and He will help me stay safe from you. So go ahead and move forward, find someone else, hopefully someone who won't abuse you like I did. Forget about me. I am not the one for you. I can't handle you anymore. I want my life back, my values and my morals. I will be the mother and friend and sister and daughter that I used to be. Maybe even better because of all I have been through. This decision is final. There is no negotiation. If I am faced by you in the future, be aware that I will be much stronger than you have ever seen. I will be able to resist you. So don't even try. Actually, you may not even recognize me. I look and act so differently when I am not with you. It's a much better look and I am a much better woman without you. I will have so many people in my corner helping me squash any thoughts of reconciling with you. A single phone call to one of those people might be all I need to turn you down and realize how ridiculous the idea of seeing you again is. But if one phone call isn't enough, imagine that I can go find an entire room full of people that will help me fight you—and we will win. There is power in numbers. I will be surrounded by people, unlike when I was with you. I will be honest, unlike when I was with you. I will be giving and helpful to others, unlike when I was with you. I will make decisions carefully, unlike when I was with you. I will feel worthy of a good life, unlike when I was with you. Someday I may have a romantic relationship—a healthy one in which you will have no involvement. I have learned that you are such a detriment to all relationships in my life. It's not your fault but mine. I want and need a fresh start and a better existence. I want to make a difference and be the person I know I can be. But I can't do that with you. I loved you so. I will always have a very healthy respect for you. Goodbye Forever.

Karla

Step Two

"Came to believe that a Power greater than ourselves could restore us to sanity"

Obviously, my attempts at running my own life had led to disaster. It was finally clear that I could not do this on my own. My efforts at controlling my drinking, controlling situations and outcomes over which I had no control, and even the most basic skills involving caring for myself and those I loved had failed miserably. I was ready to admit that I needed help.

Step Two can be interpreted as realizing that there is a higher power in control of life, and that it is not any single human being. Some are keenly aware of what, or who, their own higher power is. Others get really hung up on this Step due to agnosticism, or atheism, or disgust for organized religion, or a host of other reasons.

For me, this Step was fairly natural. I believed fully in a God, as I understood him. I have never bought into organized religion completely, nor do I believe that every word in the Bible is truly God's word as it has been written and translated repeatedly by human beings, and therefore is subject to human error. Often people will quote scripture to attempt to prove a point. Another person can find a different passage within the same book, to attempt to disprove the first person's point. Frequently, things are taken out of context, in my experience. Again, subject to human error and interpretation.

I have heard it said that "A religious person will do what he is told, no matter what is right, whereas a spiritual person will do what is right, no matter what he is told." I have also heard it said that "religion is for people who don't want to go to hell and spirituality is for those who have already been there." I believe these sentiments are fitting for me. I am not at all saying that if you are devoutly religious that you are wrong or your motives are false, not at all! For me, I needed to first repair my spirituality, my own personal relationship with the God of my understanding. Instead of putting on a show of attending church services regularly, jumping into music performance, volunteering or whatever host of other ways to "show" that I was becoming spiritual. That would have been the exact thing I was trying to get away from. It had to be about me, renewing my own personal spirituality with God and the world. I needed genuine and private spirituality. It couldn't be about me putting on airs for God or anyone else.

For me, Step Two came down to realizing that I needed help and there were people out there to help me as well as my own personal forgiving and gracious God who, in my belief, had been there all the time waiting me to begin to rely on Him again. But, even if I hadn't had that relationship and belief, I have eyes. I could look back and see my life for what it had become—a complete and utter mess. I could look at the beauty of the world around me, the oceans and lakes, mountains, sunrise and sunset, and realize that no human power created this. In fact, humans have done a bang up job of trying to destroy this beauty.

Also, as a medical provider, I was in awe of the human body and became convinced during gross anatomy lab that human beings were not just accidentally here. The way we are put together, the way all systems work in harmony when someone is healthy, the blood and the digestion and the amazing brain. That is beyond human creation, in my opinion.

As I sat in the groups and spent hour after hour with Sam, I also became aware that the community of people in recovery was also a higher power for me. Here was a group of people who, outside of addiction, often had little in common. Yet, we all were there together, supporting each other and listening to each other, trying to help one another navigate this new and scary territory. The higher power of the fellowship of people in recovery has become stronger for me with each passing year, as I have now developed real relationships with people. I have accountability within the groups that I am a part of. If I don't show up, people worry and call me out. There an understanding and acceptance within my recovery groups that is almost palpable to me.

I knew I was ready to accept help from counselors, doctors, colleagues, friends, family, others in recovery, and my God. I had felt like such a crappy human for so long that I had begun to hide from even Him. Praying felt impossible because I had so many past deeds I was ashamed of, that asking for forgiveness seemed crazy. But clear headed and beginning a true program of recovery, I could let the love in, from Him and from so many others. I came to believe in several powers greater than myself.

Step Three

"Made a decision to turn our will and our lives over to the care of God as we understood Him"

"Thy will, not mine, be done," is one of the many sayings in recovery. For me personally, this is the absolute best way to summarize Step Three. I have friends in recovery that do not believe in any god or specific higher power entity, but believe in the fellowship of recovery groups. For them, they often rely more on the saying "do the next right thing." In yet other words, as written on page 60 of the Big Book of Alcoholics Anonymous "The first requirement is that we be convinced that any life run on self-will can hardly be a success."

I learned that having attempted my entire life to control more than just me, my actions, and my reactions—I had set myself up for crushing blows, disappointments, sadness, and of course, addiction. In trying to act perfect, look perfect, BE perfect, I then expected to be appreciated for that. When I wasn't, I was let down. When I was let down, I drank. I had been manipulative with avoidance and chameleon-like behavior, which I did not realize until recovery. I had worked my ass off for many things, and been rewarded sometimes, but not others. Those times when I didn't feel that I had been treated fairly, or gotten the raise I deserved or the respect I craved, I took it so very personally. When I planned the perfect dinner party, for example, down to making twenty-three from scratch fancy appetizers and having every drink and dessert possible and the house decorated impeccably—I waited for the guests and craved their praise. If someone did not have a wonderful time, I tried to "make" them have a good time and cater to them specifically. If I didn't get compliments, I felt resentful. I wanted people to appreciate my efforts. When they didn't do so to my liking, I felt hurt and angry. I began to learn by taking Step Three that I needed to check my motives. Why had I done all of that? For attention and praise because my own feelings of self- worth were so poor that I needed it from other people. From then on, I tried to focus on why I was doing something. Focus on the effort but then realize that the outcome was not at all in my hands.

It is hard to mess with perfection, so I will quote yet another passage from the Big Book relating to Step Three which describes my past life to the letter. "Each person is like an actor who wants to run the whole show; is forever trying to arrange the lights, the ballet, the scenery and the rest of the players in his own way. If his arrangements would only stay put, if only people would do as he wished, the show would be great. Everybody, including himself, would be pleased. Life would be wonderful. In trying to make these arrangements our actor may sometimes be quite virtuous. He may be kind, considerate, patient, generous; even modest and self-sacrificing. On the other hand, he may be mean, egotistical, selfish and dishonest. But, as with most humans, he is more likely to have varied traits. What usually happens? The show doesn't come off very well. He begins to think life doesn't treat him right. He decides to exert himself more. He becomes, on the next occasion, still more demanding or gracious, as the case may be. Still, the play does not suit him. Admitting he may be somewhat at fault, he is sure that other people are more to blame. He becomes angry, indignant, self-pitying. What is his basic trouble? Is he not really a self-seeker even when trying to be kind? Is he not a victim of the delusion that he can wrest satisfaction and happiness out of this world if he only manages well?"

That was me. Trying to run the show. Trying to be in control of things I had no business trying to control. Even though I felt, at the time, that I was doing the right thing and being a good person, I was really just a scared little girl desperate for love, approval, attention and praise because I did not feel good enough about myself on my own.

Step Three is a daily challenge for me. Often I catch myself in old patterns and try to work quickly to check my motives and reroute if necessary. I find myself looking towards the sky and chanting "Thy will, not mine, Thy will, not mine, Thy will, not mine." Most of the time, it works. Sometimes, my old patterns get in the way and I make stupid choices and wind up resentful and hurt. But, it is much, much better.

Step Four

"Made a searching and fearless moral inventory of ourselves"

Step Four was the turning point for me. My counselor, Sam, walked me through how to do this searching and fearless moral inventory. The idea was frightening. I had to look at my entire past and write down my actions, what I did, who I wronged, who I thought wronged me, my resentments, my patterns in life up to that point. The task was daunting and I was exhausted just thinking about embarking upon it. There was so much that I was ashamed of. I was hurt and frail and scared. But, I did it.

My first Fourth Step with Sam, in hand written words, was 106 pages long. As a hilarious speaker at a recovery meeting once said, "All my life, I had thought I was a good person. Within my Fourth Step, I could find NO evidence to support that." How true! I wrote and wrote, listing my flaws and consequences, harms and resentments, and my part in each of the harms and resentments. With each past deed, I also needed to sort out why I had behaved the way I had. Was it fear? Trust issues? Poor self-esteem or pride run wild? Was I searching for love or security?

There were twenty-five people or entities on my resentment list. Of course the obvious, like my ex-husband, my sister, my parents. Also, my previous employer, HPSP, and the Board of Medical Practice. I was upset with so many people and things, and Sam forced me to realize and write down my part in creating the mess, situation, or resentment. That was very challenging. It was not easy to look at myself with such clarity and truth. But it was critical to my recovery. There was no way for me to move ahead with an authentic and genuine life in sobriety without first facing what I had done in the past, and more importantly, figure out why I had done the things I had. One of the most astounding realizations I made during this process was that the majority of resentments that I had involving my loved ones were because of things they had done to try to stop me from drinking. Why had they done that? *Because they loved me.* I was holding onto resentments because people loved me!! All my life, working so hard to be loved, and these people had bent over backwards to try to love me and keep me alive, and I was mad at them! Wow. What a fool I was. Once I realized this, those resentments melted away in an instant.

In my opinion, everyone should do a Fourth Step, not just addicts and alcoholics. It was cathartic, like a major case of the stomach flu. Sins and fears and experiences and anger all came rushing out of me. It took me a whole week of writing almost non-stop to complete it. Sam allowed me to miss some groups to continue to write. I was reliving my past, feeling it, breathing it, dreaming about it, and having nightmares and flashbacks. I dredged up things I hadn't even thought about in years. It was indeed a searching and fearless moral inventory.

The vast majority of my resentments and harms were related to fear and pride. Pride? Seriously? I felt like I had been a modest and gracious person. Perhaps on the outside, but inside my pride was running rampant and my fears were driving my life. Fear of withdrawal of love, fear of people not liking me, fear of failure, fear of abandonment, fear of people in general, fear of financial ruin, fear of not being good enough, fear fear fear!! And the reason my pride was off the charts was because I equated success and perfection with being loved. If I succeeded and was perfect, people would love me. If I wasn't perfect, or God forbid failed, they wouldn't. I had been leading a life so full of fear that I could no longer see reality. My perceptions had become warped. I barely knew who I was anymore.

Because of fear, I had become dishonest to the point that lying was second nature- knee jerk, even about the silliest things. I was selfish. I manipulated. I drank to relieve my fear. Little by little, I became unrecognizable inside. My motives had been pure at first, I just wanted to be loved and needed and respected. But I had gone about it all wrong. I realized that for my entire life I had been searching for peace and serenity, and all along it had actually been ME causing the chaos and anxiety I was so desperate to be rid of. What a concept! *I* had screwed up my life. *Me*. Nobody else. Me.

Holy shit.

Step Five

"Admitted to God, to ourselves, and to another human being the exact nature of our wrongs"

It was one thing to write down a lifetime of situations and events that filled me with shame. In Step Five, I had to tell all of this to another human being. Oh. My. God. For someone who always wanted everyone to like me, spilling my deepest darkest secrets to Sam (someone I now respected and who I really, REALLY wanted to like me) scared the crap out of me. Literally. I had diarrhea leading up to our first session of Fifth Step work! Too much information? Probably.

Over the next two weeks, Sam spent twenty hours with me listening to my Fifth Step. He asked questions and helped me sort through the underlying reasons for my actions and feelings. He challenged and pushed me. He was always kind.

The first session, I lied to him. I left out a very critical issue. I was too afraid to tell him because I didn't want him to think less of me. What a huge ego I had! There I was, in rehab, having blown up my life, and I was worried about what my counselor might think of me! Having returned to my room after the session and spending some time thinking, I made the decision to go back the next day and tell him I lied. I had to start being truly honest or this was never going to work. The nagging feeling in the pit of my stomach told me that I had to come clean and that I could not start off recovery based upon any more lies, or I would just build up my house of cards again—which would be sure to fall down in record speed.

From then on, I was honest with Sam. Painfully, brutally honest. Through this process, I learned about my patterns and my defaults, my strengths and my flaws. I did not realize at the time, but Sam was making my fourth and Fifth Step also encompass Steps Six, Seven and Eight. I found that if you do a thorough job on Step Four, those next action Steps came almost naturally. I cried, I was angry, I was sad and I was frustrated. Little by little, I felt the weight of the world falling off of my shoulders. I felt lighter in spirit and body. I felt like I could do this and I became convinced that recovery was possible and I could have a great, honest life. I was finding the peace and serenity I had craved my entire life. My relationship with God was becoming stronger because I felt a great sense of relief through my confessions to Sam. Ironically, I felt strength and power from admitting my powerlessness over alcohol. I had lived in the problem of alcoholism for so long that I didn't know any other life or that a different kind of life was even possible. I had begun to live in the solution of recovery and it felt amazing and I felt hopeful for my future. I knew what the damn problem was—and I was starting to grasp the way to fix it!

The cravings for the drink began to fade about halfway through my Fifth Step. I noticed that I had stopped trying to outsmart the system. I was not looking for a way to escape and run to the liquor store. I was not scheming how I could still get by with drinking and just try to control it better when I got home. I had become convinced that my life was worth living without drinking. For years I had been frightened that if I stopped drinking, I would no longer have fun. I honestly hadn't known what the point of going through life sober would be. In the past when people would tell me they didn't drink, my secret reaction was *"why on earth not"?* I thought they were crazy, they clearly didn't know what they were missing out on! I was beginning to understand. Hallelujah!

There is a story, about a hopeless drunk who had somehow ended up in a deep hole by the side of the road. People saw him and tried to figure out how to help this poor soul. Some gave him food, which he ate, but he could not get out of the pit. Others provided him money, which he then used to have still others buy him more alcohol. A priest handed him a bible to read. He read it, but still was stuck. On and on, the people looked down at him, threw scraps of wisdom, advice, monetary goods, and sometimes just looked at him with disgust and confusion. The man became seemingly permanently planted in his hole. Then one day, another man stopped, looked at him with his mouth agape, and jumped right down in that hole too. The drunk exclaimed "what are you doing, you fool? Now we are both stuck in this hole!" The other man said "Oh, it's

OK. I've been here before and I know the way out." That was Sam. He knew the way out of the pit of despair because he had been in that very same pit and escaped. Thank God for Sam!

Step Six

"Were entirely ready to have God remove all these defects of character"

During treatment, I worked Steps Six and Seven fairly quickly and alone in my room. These are reflective Steps, during which I figured out what my problems were and worked to become more aware of those flaws and how to stop myself from making the same mistakes. I was convinced that I wanted to remain sober and I was willing to do anything required, including changing myself.

I worked Step Six much more thoroughly with my sponsor, Judy, about a year into recovery. We spent almost an entire year on them. I think Steps Six and Seven are underrated Steps and actually were quite critical in maintaining happiness and sobriety for me. Judy and I read the book "Drop the Rock" and it's follow up book by Fred Holmquist "The Ripple Effect." Out loud we read these books. We dug very deeply into my character flaws.

My biggest issues had been dishonesty, self-will, overabundant pride, self-hate, selfishness, and fear. I also struggled to a slightly lesser degree with unreasonable expectations, manipulative behavior, isolation tendencies, and self-sabotage. Some flaws had only reared their ugly heads towards the end of my active addiction, and those that had always been there had been clearly exaggerated by alcoholism. Sam and later my sponsor Judy both encouraged me to aim for stabilization of these flaws, or even to attempt to veer more towards the opposite of them. Character defects are often innate, second nature, and very challenging to truly change. It is possible, however, to manage them. Some had only really become apparent during my addiction. It was first necessary to become aware that I even had defects of character, which was the whole point of Step Six.

The opposite of dishonesty obviously is honesty and that was my goal. The opposite of self-will is Thy will. The opposite of perfectionism is acceptance. The opposite of overabundant pride is to be humble and to have humility. The opposite of selfishness is selflessness. The opposite of fear is a healthy enough self-esteem and self-confidence that I could trust and rely on myself enough to handle things that I feared in a rational and reasonable manner, with perspective.

It seemed that I needed to entirely change who I had become. Stopping drinking had been, of course, necessary. But that alone would not provide happiness, and without happiness, how could I expect to stay sober? I needed to learn to be honest, rely on God and others, have humility, be selfless, and begin to have self-esteem and self-confidence. Was that even possible for me? It seemed doubtful, but I was ready to try. To have even the smallest chance of success, however, I was going to need help—a LOT of help.

Step Seven

"Humbly asked Him to remove our shortcomings"

Hooray! I knew what my problems were. Now I just needed to get rid of those flaws. On paper, it was easy, in practice, not so much. I wanted to be a better person, a whole person who treated me and other people well. I wanted healthy relationships. I wanted to make amends for all of my past deeds, but was learning that when there had been months or years of damage done to people, amends were going to take time. Many of the people I had hurt were not ready to hear apologies from me. My words did not mean much, and rightly so, as the majority of what had come out of my mouth during the past year had been lies. Those loved ones were going to need time to watch and see if I could stay sober. Trust had been broken and if it was ever going to be repaired, it had to be on their timeline.

I had to focus on me. I read about Step Seven in the Big Book and it recommended that once an alcoholic has become aware of their character flaws and become ready to rid themselves of those flaws that they move ahead to Step Seven. The weird thing is, my old ways were what I knew. If I changed dramatically, who would I really be? Was I going to lose myself further by attempting such a complete turnabout? There was fear of the unknown. I finally realized that even though the future me was a work in progress and the outcome unknown, I knew without a doubt that I no longer wanted to be the person I had become. I was ready.

To do so, I needed to pray to my higher power and ask Him to remove my shortcomings. A recommended prayer on page seventy-six of the Big Book follows.

"My Creator, I am now willing that you should have all of me, good and bad. I pray that you now remove from me every single defect of character which stands in the way of my usefulness to you and my fellows. Grant me strength, as I go out from here, to do your bidding. Amen."

In my room, I quietly said this prayer—twice, in fact. The first time through, I felt kind of silly and awkward. I realized I hadn't really said the words with meaning or intent, but just simply read them. I took a few deep breaths and did it again but much slower, stopping after each phrase to really absorb the seriousness and magnitude of what I was saying.

Next, I wrote it down in my own words, potty mouth and all. "My God, Please take all of me; all of my shit and all of my goodness. Take away all of these messed up character flaws I have and help me treat everyone, including myself, the way they deserve to be treated. Be with me as I move forward, because I am scared to death and I know I can't do it without You. Thy will, not mine, be done."

The relief was instant. I FELT that I was no longer alone. I KNEW that I would always have help to do the next right thing. I felt a sense of peace that is beyond words. When I tried to tell Sam of this experience, his joyful smile revealed that he knew exactly of what I spoke because he had been there.

Step Eight

"Made a list of all persons we had harmed, and became willing to make amends to them all"

Holy crap. When done correctly, this Step is as fearless and searching as the Fourth Step. In fact, my Eighth Step was nearly complete because I had done my Fourth Step so thoroughly. I already had listed the harms I had caused and the resentments I held as well as my part in any conflict. I had a very complete list of twenty-five people and groups, with all of the yucky details about what I had done. There were only two situations/people that both Sam and my sponsor agreed would result in more hurt to them or others if an amends was made, but everyone else I was going to have to face in due time. I was fully aware of my past actions and the destruction I had caused. I wanted very badly to make things right. I wanted it immediately, in fact. But as I stated in Step Seven, I would have to wait. Words were useless that early in recovery. Of course I was still sober—I was locked up! The real test would be once I had been back in the real world for a while. They would need to watch how I acted, what I did, how I handled issues, and if I could stay away from the booze. Sixty-four days may have seemed fairly lengthy to me but for them, it was just a reprieve from dealing with my bullshit and knowing I was safe in a facility. Their fear for the future was enormous and justified; their doubt evident and their distrust so obvious. I had a lot of work to do. I had to learn patience, and that time was my friend.

One of my very favorite passages in the Big Book relating to the loved ones of an alcoholic is on page eighty-two. "The alcoholic is like a tornado roaring his way through the lives of others. Hearts are broken. Sweet relationships are dead. Affections have been uprooted. Selfish and inconsiderate habits have kept the home in turmoil. We feel a man is unthinking when he says that sobriety is enough. He is like the farmer who came up out of his cyclone cellar to find his home ruined. To his wife, he remarked, "Don't see anything the matter here, Ma. Ain't it grand the wind stopped blowin?" This passage is no more ridiculous than me thinking that everything should be fine and forgiven now that I stopped drinking.

Stopping drinking was just the beginning. It was necessary, of course, but being dry was not the end all by any means. Time was required to establish new habits and behaviors, to rebuild the wreckage of my life, to clean my side of the street and start anew. Alcoholics desire instant gratification. Drinking provides near immediate relief for the drunk. I had relied on it for years to squash my feelings of discomfort, unease, anxiety, sadness, even happiness. I drank to numb the bad things, but inadvertently ended up numbing everything—including happiness. I was going to have to learn to sit with my feelings, learn to be uncomfortable, sad, or uneasy and deal with that in ways other than the instant relief of alcohol. For me to sit patiently and just keep slowly and routinely doing the right things, was extremely challenging. Sometimes I was so tempted to call people and try to push or even force my way back into their lives, to tell on the mountain how I had changed and that all should be forgiven.

Sam, of course, understood that impatience and frustration. He knew the desire to right the wrongs RIGHT NOW DAMN IT!! But he explained to me that while I had been focusing on my recovery and making huge changes to myself, those I had hurt were still just reeling from the past and trying to catch their balance. They were not ready for me, they may never be, and I could not run my recovery and life hoping to impress others or regain their love. I had to run my recovery to stay sober and find personal fulfillment and contentment. It was NOT contingent upon their forgiveness or love. Coming to terms with the fact that some of the damage I had done may be permanent was not easy. But I did learn to accept it, and to hand this, along with everything else, to my Higher Power. I could put forth all of the effort I needed and feel good about that, but the outcome was not in my hands. Nor had it ever been, actually. I was only responsible for my expectations, actions, and reactions. I had no control over the expectations, actions, and reactions of anyone else no matter how much I had previously thought that I did.

Step Nine

"Made direct amends to such people whenever possible, except when to do so would injure them or others"

Making amends, for me, was a slow and long process. Sam talked a lot about living amends. He suggested with many of my loved ones that I make my amends by showing them, over time, that I had changed. He said that kind of amends is the most powerful and effective. He did not recommend that I begin calling people to apologize; he recommended in-person amends when possible, but that for the majority of people on my list, I was going to simply have to wait until they were ready. *If they were ever ready.*

I celebrated five years of sobriety just before writing this book. During those five years, at various times I have sat down with my parents, sister, best friend, other girlfriends, children, even my ex-husband Jim, and discussed all that I put them through. I apologized, and the amends were always extremely well received. Because I had waited and shown them for a while that I truly had changed and was sober and that I was very sorry for the harm I had caused and was doing everything in my power to ensure that it never happened again.

I finally reached out in writing to the last two people on my amends list just before my five-year sobriety anniversary. Not the people that I had been told not to make amends to, but the last two people still on the list. One did not respond. The other wrote back a fairly scathing response including that "this apology is six years too late." That stung, and required a lot of self- reflection and discussion with my sponsor and peers in my meetings. I was asked about my motives when reaching out to those last two people, because my reaction revealed that I had perhaps been truly looking for absolution. They were right—I had. That is NOT what an amends is about. You do not go into an amends and apologize and come clean hoping for any absolution or any type of response. You are to admit all of your sins, apologize, and whatever happens, happens. The idea is to put forth a genuine and honest amends. It is to give the person you have harmed a chance to respond, in whatever manner they need to. I realized that I had hurt this person a lot more than I even had imagined, and his response to me was as it should have been—his true honest feelings were that he was still very angry and hurt. My amends gave him a platform to express his feelings. Yes, I was hurt and sad for a while, but this was not supposed to be about me or my feelings. It was about his. So I did what did not come naturally—I simply accepted his response with a "thank you for your response, I am so sorry that I caused you so much pain." Then I let it go. The old me wanted to dig in and defend myself and give excuses for my behavior and point out HIS issues, HIS part in the problem, HIS flaws, how HE had not been perfect either and blah blah blah. But I didn't. You know what? It feels pretty good to be able to now be at peace with it. Maybe I can become an adult after all!

My absolute favorite passage in the Big Book is called, by many in recovery, the Promises. It is on pages eighty-three and eighty-four, following instructions on how to work the Ninth Step.

"If we are painstaking about this phase of our development, we will be amazed before we are half way through. We are going to know a new freedom and a new happiness. We will not regret the past nor wish to shut the door on it. We will comprehend the word serenity and we will know peace. No matter how far down the scale we have gone, we will see how our experience can benefit others. That feeling of uselessness and self-pity will disappear. We will lose interest in selfish things and gain interest in our fellows. Self-seeking will slip away. Our whole attitude and outlook upon life will change. Fear of people and of economic insecurity will leave us. We will intuitively know how to handle situations which used to baffle us. We will suddenly realize that God is doing for us what we could not do for ourselves. Are these extravagant promises? We think not. They are being fulfilled among us—sometimes quickly, sometimes slowly. They will always materialize if we work for them."

The first time I heard the promises, way back in Hazelden, I thought *"bullshit."* Part way through my stay at the Recovery Village, working the Steps with Sam, I thought *"maybe there is some truth to these Promises."* And now, five years sober, they have ALL come true. No shit.

Step Ten

"Continued to take personal inventory and when we were wrong promptly admitted it"

Taking the Steps the first time was exhausting but necessary. Thirty-nine years of harms and resentments, reliving situations that were not pleasant, apologizing and digging in deep into my character flaws required a lot of time and energy. I never wanted to rack up that many years of misdeeds and mistakes again! Thus began the maintenance Steps.

Steps One, Two, and Three were really all about surrender. I don't care for the term because to me it sounds like giving up, which was the opposite of what I was doing. Surrender, however, is the term accepted by most people in recovery to explain the moment when they realized that their addiction was smarter than they were and was going to kill them if they did not take action. So, I feel more like it was the moment in which *I decided* I could no longer drink and I was ready and willing to do anything I had to. Even if that meant letting go of my supposed control, going through a painful recap of my history, and apologizing to people for horrendous acts I had committed that I would have preferred to pretend never happened.

Steps Four, Five, Six, Seven and Eight were action Steps—requiring me to do a lot of work, some of which was very difficult. So, after surrendering to alcoholism, and reconnecting with my Higher Power, and after doing all of the work of reviewing my past and making amends, it was time to learn about the maintenance steps.

I really wanted to know how I could avoid creating another 106 page novel about bad shit I did. I did NOT want a sequel to that. The Tenth Step is really important in preventing history from repeating itself. Done on a daily basis, it is much more manageable than trying to tackle thirty-nine years at once. The Tenth Step is all about truly thinking about each day as it comes to a close. Did I say or do anything harmful today? Do I need to make amends to anyone for things I did? Did I notice any or all of my character defects popping out? If so, what am I going to do about it?

I find if I do this every night, and follow through the next day with making right anything that I need to, I continue to feel the lightness and peace that flooded me following my Fourth and Fifth Step. If I let too many days go by without doing a Tenth Step, things begin to build up and procrastination can creep in. That is a slippery slope for me. My anxiety builds and fear tries to take over my life. When I am fearful, all of my character defects of dishonesty and manipulation and everything else start to kick in again. I feel myself becoming irritated easily, restless and discontent. The easiest way I know to relieve myself of those uncomfortable feelings, of course, is to drink which I no longer do. So, I have to keep a daily check on myself.

Some people do a written Tenth Step, some start by doing one every night over the phone with their sponsor, some do it with meditation or prayer, either out loud or silently in their head. It does not seem to matter how one does it, but it absolutely matters if one does not do it at all. Not keeping a daily check on myself is a recipe for relapse. So I do it—every night.

To help me solidify what my place is in this world, what I have control over, what I don't, and whether or not I have done things or reacted in ways that I shouldn't have on any given day, I rely on the principles of the book "The Four Agreements." Anyone in recovery absolutely should read and re-read this book, in my opinion. Actually, anyone who is alive should read it. Having not asked for permission to disclose snippets of "The Four Agreements," I will say nothing more except that it has been a Godsend to me and I recommend it highly.

Step Eleven

"Sought through prayer and meditation to improve our conscious contact with God as we understood Him, praying only for knowledge of His will for us and the power to carry that out"

Step Eleven, for me, is about keeping the faith, and praying every morning for strength and wisdom to do what is right. I also ask for help to stay sober. I thank my higher power for all that I have to be grateful for and ask for continued help to do His will, rather than mine. You don't have to pray, if you aren't into that. You can simply read your gratitude list and asset list to start the day off with a firm grasp on reality. You can call your sponsor or send a text with a message that you are grateful to be sober. I do pray, because that works for me, but don't let the God language turn you off of this Step because it is truly about gratitude and perspective in my opinion—and is not a Step to be overlooked.

Sam assigned me the task of writing an all-encompassing gratitude list and asset list. These I began in treatment, and I continue to add to them—especially the gratitude list. Including even things such as indoor plumbing and electricity, along with the more obvious things such as my children, has been very good for me. I needed to put things in perspective. Yes, I had wrecked my life, but there in treatment in a warm room with plenty of food and luxuries, my life was still a hell of a lot better than many in the world. I had to keep that in mind. It would have been easy to throw myself a pity party on a regular basis and focus on what I had lost—and believe me, I had those moments. But I focused daily on what I DID have, the blessings in my life, the hope for my future. These kept me in a better state of mind and connected with reality.

And the reality is, I am blessed. The majority of people in this country have opportunities, help (yes, you have to ask for it), welfare (yes, you may have to humble yourself enough to sit in a crowded welfare office all day and tell your story to the social worker), medical options (again, you have to humble yourself and sign up for the free or reduced cost care), bountiful food (yes, you might have to go to a shelter or food shelf if you are hard up but it's there to be had). We are not, in this country, grasping for a grain of rice. I am sure there are exceptions, and I apologize if I have offended anyone, but I have found that all of my needs can easily be met in the USA, if I put my tail between my legs and just admit I need help. Alcoholics, by nature, are not good at that. Go back to Step One if you really think you don't need any help.

Over the years, my gratitude list has grown exponentially. It would take several pages in this book if I were to list all that I have to be grateful for. It is empowering to look at that every morning and see how things just continue to improve the longer I am sober. Is that because I am more aware of my blessings? Or is it that through sobriety I have been granted more and more blessings over time? I think both. I don't believe I would ever be this grateful, happy, and fulfilled had I not gone through my alcoholism and subsequent crash. But the biggest change is that I continually work the Steps, which keeps me humble and keeps things in perspective. I am simply a much better person because I am in recovery. I actually like me now!

When I first went to treatment back at Hazelden, some of the old timers in the program would call themselves "grateful recovering alcoholics." I cringed and shook my head every time I heard it. What the hell is there to be grateful for here? I don't want to be an alcoholic. I don't want to stop drinking! I want to be just like other people! I want my old life back! This crap is bullshit! Let me out of here! You people are crazy!

Guess what? Now *I am* a grateful recovering alcoholic.

Step Twelve

"Having had a spiritual awakening as the result of these Steps, we tried to carry this message to alcoholics and to practice these principles in all our affairs"

Helping others helps me. It is quite a concept. I love Step Twelve so much that I very easily could have been a "two-stepper," which refers to people who only work Step One and Step Twelve. But, Sam, and later my sponsor Judy, made it crystal clear that two-steppers don't typically achieve long-term sobriety—those other Steps two through eleven are in the Big Book for very important reasons. How very glad I am for their guidance, then and now.

Step Twelve is about giving back the wisdom you have accumulated, and sharing your experience, strength, and hope with others who desire sobriety. This started out for me by being an honest participant in groups while in treatment, then by helping to make coffee or bring some cookies for a meeting. Driving others to and from meetings is also Twelfth Step work.

Once home, I also took on a role as a "trusted servant" for a month at a meeting I liked, meaning I would lead the meeting each week for that month. Eventually, I began speaking at other meetings, even going back up to Hazelden to speak to their health care group. I would go with my sponsor or with others to local treatment centers to share my story. Continually exposing myself to those brand new to recovery, or those back in treatment for the twentieth time provided a keen awareness as to what I would be facing if I chose to drink again. If I ever was having a day where I felt either over-confident about my recovery, or on the flip side, depressed or "poor-me", going to one of those meetings and seeing the fear, the disgrace, the shame on the faces put me right back on track.

A chiropractor in recovery and a dear friend of mine, Lisa, wanted to initiate a health care provider recovery meeting in our area, as the nearest one was about an hour away. She did not want to undertake this on her own and was looking for a partner. After some thought, I agreed to help. This meeting has been in place for over three years, continues to grow (we even had to relocate the meeting to a place with more space), and is my favorite hour of the week most of the time. Lisa has since bowed out to pursue more Big Book studies, but I attend it faithfully almost every week. Hazelden sends some of their patients who work in healthcare to us each week, so we are frequently seeing new people. Our core group continues to grow, and now even HPSP (the state healthcare provider monitoring agency) recommends our meeting to their participants. It's a really cool thing and it helps a great deal in keeping me sober.

My sponsor, Judy, recommended I do some work bringing recovery meetings into the Washington County Jail. I was pretty frightened about this, as I had never spent any time in jail, though God knows I could have and probably should have been there many, many times. There was some training for this, including boundaries and guidelines as well as a tour. The locking doors and lack of buttons in elevators and massive security were shocking for me and gave me another huge reason to be grateful that I had not wound up in there. We read parts of the Big Book, and also stories from a terrific book called "Inmate to Inmate." Going to the jail to share my story and listen to the stories of other women addicts and alcoholics who are facing serious prison time or skid row if they are released, was the best advice I have received to date from my sponsor.

If someone is struggling with their active addiction and calls me, I pick up. If someone else asks if I will call a person in the program who is struggling, I call. A person working a true program of recovery will always find the time and energy to help someone else struggling with addiction who is asking for help.

It's a weird thing that doing Twelve-Step work actually helps the person providing the help often more than the person receiving. I think this is how and why the program works. It's a continuous cycle of old timers and newcomers, the old timers with a breadth of wisdom, the newcomers laden with such hopelessness and shame. It reminds the old timers of where they don't want to ever go again while providing real hope for the newcomers that there is the possibility of a great life in recovery.

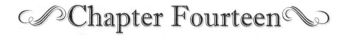Chapter Fourteen

SPONSORSHIP

Probably one of the most important components of Twelve-Step work, if not THE most important, is sponsorship. Both having a sponsor and later becoming a sponsor have been instrumental in my recovery. A sponsor is someone with some recovery time under their belt, who helps a newcomer or someone else within the program navigate life sober. I think the term "mentor" is a bit better fit, but who am I to attempt to change several decades of recovery terminology?

Sam encouraged me to find a sponsor right away upon returning home. Often, the first sponsor you have is really a temporary one to help you until you find someone who has what you want and you ask them to become your permanent sponsor. Those is sort of the loose guideline—look around the rooms and observe, watch for someone who seems to have what you want in terms of life, happiness, personality and ask them.

I got lucky because the first person I noticed was a woman named Judy. She had eight years sober. I couldn't imagine eight months sober, eight years seemed incredible. She had gotten sober when her two kids, a boy and a girl, were eight and ten, almost the same ages as mine were at the time I left inpatient treatment. Judy was glowing. She was happy, and funny; smart and charming. But she was also honest and not afraid to tell her story. Looking at her, I could really not imagine that this put together calm and lovely woman had ever been completely and hopelessly addicted to alcohol. But she had been. And she had gotten through it!!

I asked her to be my sponsor. That is hard to do, asking someone to commit to helping you on a one to one basis, for potentially a lifetime. She had what I could only dream of having, but wanted. She said yes! We met every single week for up to three hours each time. I told her my story; she told me parts of hers. I worked the Steps with her in a much more meticulous and slow manner now that it was my second time working them. I redid my Fourth Step and told it to her in my Fifth Step. She did not judge, she still seemed to like me, and she offered sound advice when I asked for it.

She helped me get through all of my amends. She picked up the phone anytime I called, and was quick to reach out to me if she hadn't heard from me for a bit. Not only is she my sponsor, but she is one of my very best friends and someone I admire immensely. Anytime that I am struggling with a decision or something challenging that I am facing, or something that I am simply scared to death about, Judy is there. When things are going well, she is there. She is very supportive and helpful, but never tells me what to do. She helps me work through my motives, fears, successes and helps me to figure things out for myself. When I make a mistake, she helps me right it. But never judges me. I trust her implicitly.

About two years into recovery, someone asked me to be their sponsor. I was unsure, I didn't feel ready. My sponsor told me I was more than ready and encouraged me to accept the role and the challenges that would come with it. So I did. My first sponsee was a woman named Heather. She was a chronic relapser, having been in and out of the program for quite some time. She was facing serious consequences from her alcoholism and really wanted to be sober. I was hopeful that I could help. I tried to give her the same patience and understanding that had been given to me. I tried to make recovery related tasks less of a chore for her and more encouraging. She would stay sober for a few months, and then stop calling and stop attending meetings. Out of the blue, she would turn up again and describe her horrific recent drunken past. She would be determined to try again, and I would attempt to help her. As this pattern continued to repeat itself, I wondered if I was any good at this sponsor business, because it certainly didn't seem to be helping her. My sponsor and I decided it was actually a good test for me—to try my best but have to accept whatever outcome was to be. I couldn't be a perfectionist in this case. I couldn't base things on the outcome, which was out of my control. I couldn't take it personally if Heather stopped calling or coming, or take it as a personal failure if she did not find a happy recovery.

She ended up in rehab again and I didn't hear from her for many months, until one day she was back at the health care recovery meeting, stating that she had relapsed again but was trying so hard and had found a new sponsor. At first, I was a little hurt and wondered why I wasn't good enough. There it was—good old fear coming into play. My sponsor helped me work through it, and ultimately I was able to let it go and be at peace with it. Heather came a couple more times to that meeting, and now I haven't seen or heard from her in over six months.

My second sponsee was an RN named Nina, who had been caught tampering with pain pumps at the hospital in which she worked. She was facing criminal charges, had lost her RN license and her job, and was devastated. She was young, twenty-four. I couldn't imagine having to give up my alcohol at twenty-four, and empathized with her so much. She worked the Steps, diligently and thoroughly. We met weekly. She then met a man, became pregnant, married him, and moved several hours away. She needed to find a new sponsor and new meetings locally. To my knowledge, she is still sober and working her program, though we speak infrequently.

Lindsey was my third. Oh funny, beautiful, witty Lindsey. I took her on at the request of her father Luther, who was part of my health care recovery meeting. Lindsey had been living in San Francisco and had become heavily addicted to alcohol. She had moved back to Minnesota to try to remove herself from that lifestyle and settle down with the help of her sober father and stepmother, Dawn. Lindsey was twenty-four. Alcohol was her drug of choice. She had been adopted as an infant, and part of the reason she had gone to San Francisco had been to reconnect with her birth mother, Charity. Boy had they connected! They were like two peas in a pod. Lindsey described their time together as magical, instant bonding, and having filled a void that she hadn't even realized existed. They spent nearly every moment together. They worked together. And they drank together. Really drank. Even at their work, at a cigar shop, they drank. After work, they drank. They played board games into the night, drinking. It was beautiful—until it wasn't. She realized that she couldn't keep on with that lifestyle, and also felt that her mother, who had already been through two near fatal episodes of alcohol induced pancreatitis, also needed to slow down. Lindsey felt that if she weren't there, her mother would be less likely to drink so heavily.

So, she moved here to be with her father. I met Lindsey in June of 2017. She was so sad. She missed her mother terribly. She missed alcohol terribly. Upon arrival in Minnesota, she attended a LGBTQ (she was gay) rehab program called "Pride," where she met many friends. She became somewhat of a mother figure to several of the other clients, taking on their problems as her own. Lindsey was so caring and loving, so giving and compassionate. Their pain became hers—on top of the deep pain she already felt. We worked together, meeting every week. She could not get past Step One. I could understand this—she was so young, and leaving alcohol behind at such a young age meant also leaving her entire friend group and social circle behind. She was trying to reinvent her entire life. She sought counseling, and her counselor recommended no contact with her birth mother, at least for a while. Lindsey tried to abide by that, but simply couldn't. Her parents here tried very hard to help, to reach her, to do sober activities, to make her feel welcome and important. It felt like we were all making a bit of a difference.

On August 14, 2017, Lindsey called me at 10:30 pm. She told me she was drunk (actually, she told me in jovial laughter that she was "messed up"), and was worried her dad was going to be disappointed in her. She was parked down the street from his house, she said. I asked her what she was going to do. She told me she was going to go home and try to sneak in the house and go to sleep so she wouldn't have to face her dad and tell him she had relapsed. I told her I thought that was a good idea and that we would deal with all of it in the morning. She asked me to promise her I wouldn't "tattle" on her. As a sponsor, it is not my job to go tattling on sponsees—in fact you just don't do it unless the person is in danger of hurting themselves or others. She assured me she was not suicidal or in any danger, just drunk, and promised to go home and call me in the morning. She agreed, told me she loved me, and hung up.

Lindsey apparently did go home and sneak in. She also apparently got a phone call from an ex-girlfriend which did not go well. She apparently left the house again, continued to drink, and hung herself in the park near her father's home. Lindsey died by suicide as a direct result of her alcoholism. This disease is not a joke. It wants to kill those afflicted with it, and it got Lindsey. I had felt that helpless once before in my life, when my dear cousin Jackie died by suicide in 2012. All of the what if's, and should have's and could have's and guilt and questions and anger—it all came flooding in. The outpouring of love from Lindsey's friends and family would have shocked her, for she felt that she was undeserving and did not feel that she mattered. She did. I struggled, and still do, with what I might have done differently. Should I have called her father to tell him Lindsey was drunk? Should I have gone to her? Maybe then she would be alive. Or, maybe then she would have had a knock down drag out fight with her dad and still ended up dying by suicide making his last encounter with her horrid. I will never know how things might have played out. However, I do know that when someone is in such gut wrenching emotional pain that they simply cannot tolerate it a minute longer, nothing and nobody can stop it. I miss her. I will always miss her.

For a period of time, I thought maybe I just wasn't supposed to be a sponsor, that I wasn't good at it, that I caused more harm than good. But this was me trying to own control for things I had no control over. My sponsor helped me see that. I brought my fears and concerns to the health care recovery group, and although they empathized, they did not feel I should stop being a sponsor. They also reminded me of the hideous statistics related to success in long-term recovery. The numbers are stacked against us, folks. They told me that I had to keep trying. They asked me if I had fifty sponsees over my lifetime and only one "made it," was that still a success? Of course it was! With such poor odds, helping even one person is so valuable. So, I got back on the horse.

Zach had been a sponsee of Luther's, Lindsey's dad. Obviously, Luther needed some time, but Zach needed ongoing and immediate help as he was newly sober. We agreed to work together until Luther was back and up to working with him again. Zach was also twenty-four and gay. Typically, one sponsors only members of the same sex, to decrease any chance of crushes or romance or sexual tension clouding any issues. With Zach, that was not an issue as he was certainly not interested romantically in a middle-aged woman. A member of the health care recovery meeting, Zach was an RN who had lost his job and his license for diverting opiates. He readily admitted that he was first and foremost, however, an alcoholic, and probably had been from about the age of fifteen. He had gone so far as to never even get his driver's license because he realized that in his addicted state, he had no business driving a car and putting himself and the general population at risk. Pretty wise for a teenager, I would say.

Zach had been a childhood perfectionist, and succeeded at everything he did; top of the class, musically talented, nursing school, straight into a high paying well-respected RN position. In short order all of that was ruined, as he faced the DEA, was fired from his job, and lost his nursing license. He was possibly facing felony charges as well. Given that I had lost my PA license, had to deal with national board certification and the DEA, and lost my job in the past as well as that pesky perfectionistic trait, there was a great deal of common ground. The difference was that I was about four years ahead of him on the recovery journey and had managed to claw my way back while remaining sober. He wanted what I had. We clicked. Luther, his previous sponsor, moved to a different city and stopped attending the health care meeting with regularity, so Zach and I became "official." We meet, to this day, every week—sometimes twice. I am certain I get more out of these meetings than he does—but he likely sees it differently. I intend to work with Zach as long as he will have me, just like I intend to work with my own sponsor, Judy, as long as she will have me.

And if, or when, someone reaches out again for me, I will reach back. It's just the way it is. It is what we do.

Erik

About five weeks into treatment in Florida, my roommate Jess came into our room in the evening where I was alone as usual, reading and feverishly doing my assignments. She wanted to grab something but also wanted to tell me that there was a new guy who was from Minnesota, like me. Intrigued, I did what I rarely did in the evenings, and padded out to the common area to see what was going on. People were chatting and watching TV, some were playing games and some were outside smoking. It was comfortable chaos, but a vibe that never really interested me previously. I had been quite content to participate fully during the day in all groups, but retire after dinner to the solitude of my room to write, read, and think.

Erik was his name. And he was not at all from Minnesota; he had just attended treatment there some twelve years earlier at Hazelden. He was from Pennsylvania actually and had just transferred from an inpatient center up there. I had about five days longer sober than he did. He was a little older than me, with a thirteen year-old boy and six year-old girl and his divorce nearly finalized.

There are few times in my life that I recall such an instant connection with someone. My evening routine quickly changed entirely and I became one of the group. We sat, for three to four hours every night in two red upholstered chairs that became dubbed by the rest of the group as "ours." We laughed, we shared, and we connected. He could see how incredibly sad I was. He was confident and almost scary smart and spoke Spanish fluently. His sense of humor was killer and meshed very nicely with mine. He really listened to me. He wanted to know everything about me—my past, my future, my fears. He offered some of his past to me, and some feelings, but in hindsight, I can see that he was very cautious not to be too vulnerable. He was so incredibly supportive.

Although my focus was staying sober, things from home had to be dealt with. I would call my kids once a week. The conversations were short, and awkward, and I would be so sad afterwards. My sister was still not taking my calls, though I had received a letter from my father which was supportive, so I had some hope. I had accepted an offer on my home, which was incredible because I was very close to foreclosure. And of course, I had been dealing with the Minnesota Board of Medical Practice. I had voluntarily surrendered my license, after speaking with a wonderful woman named Ruth in that office who suggested it would be the best thing to do for the time being. To say that my future was uncertain was a huge understatement.

Erik helped me deal with all of that. He listened, he offered advice, he learned more and more about who I was and what made me tick. He became my best friend over the course of a few short days. I began to care more about my appearance. I noticed where he was and what his schedule was. I began really looking forward to our evenings in the red chairs. He was a business man, who told me of his successful equine pharmaceutical business. He had been a racehorse trainer for years, and then developed a product for GERD in racehorses that had really taken off. There were some struggles, however, between him and his co-owners. Not being a business owner, I didn't quite understand, and still don't, how that whole thing worked or what went down.

Regardless, he was yet another take-charge kind of man, smart, funny, confident; just my type. Except he wasn't angry, mean, or violent! Perhaps my tastes were changing, though my counselor Sam cautioned me heavily against pursuing anything romantic with Erik, telling me my "picker was broken." He was not pleased with this developing relationship. Sam told me he felt that Erik was exhibiting manipulative behavior and that I was searching for a partner because I had such uncertainty to go home to. He urged me to let myself be "at sea" for a while to get my bearings before tying up again at the nearest harbor. He feared we would be getting together for the wrong reasons. But that wasn't his main concern. His absolute main concern was that one of us would relapse, which almost always causes the other one to follow suit. The counselors all recommend not entering into any romantic relationships within the first year of sobriety. This was the ONLY piece of advice or recommendation from Sam that I did not follow. One would think I had learned my lesson with Mark, but in that case I hadn't actually been sober, nor had he. I truly felt this was different. Besides, I would be going back to Minnesota, and Erik back to Pennsylvania and that would likely be the end of it, so I just continued to enjoy my time with him.

One day, Sam told me he felt that I was ready to be discharged. I had told him that I was willing to stay as long as he recommended, and unlike my other rehabs, I was not marking X's on the calendar or counting any days. I was committed to staying until Sam said I didn't need to anymore. My plane ticket home was purchased, and a discharge date was set for the following week. Erik wanted to spend some time with me, on the outside, before I returned home. He checked himself out against medical advice, I changed my plane ticket for a couple of days later, and we spent two nights together in Orlando. We found meetings, we went to dinner, we talked, we made love, and we got to know each other better. I learned that Erik really didn't want to go back to Pennsylvania; he had described a tough childhood and ongoing relational issues between his parents and himself. He did not think his children were ready to see him, and his newly ex-wife did not want him back. Prior to treatment, he had packed up his belongings and placed them in a "Pod" storage unit, so he didn't even have an apartment to go to. He asked if he could come to Minnesota with me.

This felt like a lot of pressure to me, but given my fears of facing the realities at home alone, the idea of having a partner appealed to me. I gave it some deep thought and prayer over the course of those two days, and ultimately decided he could come with me.

Chapter Fifteen

RETURNING HOME

Erik and I arrived in Minnesota into one of the coldest January days on record. We were determined to succeed in our recovery, and worked as a team. We were the two musketeers! Attending at least one, if not two meetings daily became our routine. We talked, laughed, loved, and stayed sober.

I had accepted an offer on the house, and the closing was to take place three weeks after returning home. That meant that I had to sort through years of accumulated household items and memories very quickly. I had to take a loss on the house, but needed to get it sold. I simply couldn't afford it, nor did I need such a large home with all of the care it required. We found a house to rent. It seemed out of our price range, but Erik thought we would be OK. The house was beautiful, about half the size of my previous one, with gorgeous views of the St. Croix River. It was a sanctuary.

Erik took a job selling cars. I used more money from my 401K's to keep afloat. Returning to work in my trained profession would take time, if it ever were to be possible. I began teaching piano lessons intermittently to help. Food stamps and medical assistance were utilized.

Within a week of returning home, I went to Fairview to see an addiction medicine counselor to help me navigate sobriety in Minnesota. I was determined to do everything that was recommended. I was no longer trying to outsmart alcoholism and get by with shit.

I saw a counselor every week, someone recommended by Fairview. The counselor himself was in recovery, and I could not have chosen a better fit. He did not want to hear syrupy sweet things from me. He wanted the truth and knew very well when I was not being honest. He challenged me. He made other recommendations, which I followed. I saw a woman in charge of Physicians Helping Physicians in Minnesota, and also followed her recommendations. An addiction medicine physician was consulted, whom I saw, and he began providing me with monthly Vivitrol injections and encouraged continued use of Gabapentin, Trazodone, and Lexapro—all at night. Vivitrol is typically used to help those addicted to opiates. It blocks some of the opiate receptors in the brain, so that if one uses an opiate while on the Vivitrol, the effect is not realized, either with euphoria or with pain control. It had shown promise with alcoholism in studies, helping with cravings and decreasing relapse rates—though not nearly as significantly as for opiate addicts. The injection cost $1600 each time, but was mostly covered by my insurance. I wanted to have as many safeguards in place as possible, even if their success was more placebo than anything else.

I attended ninety meetings in ninety days as recommended. I found my sponsor, Judy, and began working with her in earnest almost immediately. An ignition interlock, though not court ordered, was voluntarily placed back in my car. This time, I asked that it not start if I tested over 0.00, and asked that it be tested as frequently as possible. I wanted and needed the accountability, for myself as well as in the hopes that I would eventually be allowed to see my children. I had previously "flunked out" of HPSP and surrendered my PA license, so I no longer qualified for their monitoring program. Instead, I continued to call HPSP every day and when my previous colors were called, I presented to a clinic for a self-pay observed Etg (ethyl glucuronide presence from drinking alcohol) and drug test. All of the results from the UA's and the ignition interlock were sent directly to the MN Board of Medical Practice from the companies, bypassing me in the loop to eliminate any possibility of my tampering with results. I knew that if I ever wanted to get my license back, I was going to have to prove that I was sober and safe.

Upon surrendering my license, it was relayed to me that I would not be allowed to meet with the Board or petition for a provisional PA license until I had six months of continuous sobriety, documented. The catch 22 was of course, that since I had no license I couldn't participate in the Board's monitoring program, but had to take the initiative and do it myself. None of this was inexpensive. But I was fully cognizant that without sobriety, I would have nothing else—not even my life. I continued to tap into my retirement savings to finance all of this. Recovery became my life. I read, and discussed, attended meetings, listened to audio tapes, watched "Intervention" on TV, sought out every recovery/addiction related movie I could find, dreamed it, breathed it.

Besides staying sober, I had other goals. Of course I wanted to see my children and be the mother they deserved. Reconnecting with my parents and my sister was incredibly important to me. And I wanted, and needed, to work. Preferably, in my PA career. Accepting that none of these things was going to happen quickly, if at all, was very difficult. I wanted everything back the way it had been before, except that I would be sober. I discovered how important patience in recovery was, and how difficult it was. Finding myself often having to go back to Step Three—"thy will, not mine," had become a new way of life. I was learning to accept life as it was. I continued to do everything *in my power* to do the next right thing, and slowly learned to leave the outcome of my efforts up to God. There was a huge learning curve with this, as it was totally opposite of how I had lived my life up until I got sober. In the past. I had set goals and made things happen by whatever means necessary. Letting go of supposed control was not easy for me. I say "supposed" because I really never had control but spent a lot of time trying to control things beyond my control regardless. I had to learn to continually, frequently give control to my higher power. Then I would find myself trying to take it back. It was a tug of war in my head. But as with most anything, practice helped.

Progress was painfully slow in terms of my relationships and my career. In hindsight, it is clear that the time away from work and away from my children and family was a time of immense personal growth and commitment to recovery. Had my wish of instant return to work and relationships come true, I would have been sure to relapse because I wouldn't have learned the new habits critical to long term sobriety. As much as it hurt, it was important for me to sit with my feelings and deal with my consequences. I needed to reflect and reprioritize, to pray, to establish a new normal for myself. I needed to learn to live life, complete with struggles and disappointments, without alcohol. And it was hard. There were so many times that I felt defeated, where I felt the progress was too slow and doubted if I had it in me to stay sober. Reaching for my crutch of alcohol had become so second nature, that newly sober I often would truly reach for my bottle which was not there, in an attempt to soothe my feelings. It was during these times, that my new sober network, including Erik, was lifesaving. Nobody understands this the way another alcoholic does. If I was craving a drink or feeling like I couldn't do it anymore, I certainly couldn't call my mom and vent this to her—she would have been terrified! But, I could tell Erik or Judy. Or go to a meeting and tell the whole room. And they would get it. And they would convince me to keep moving forward, yet with the understanding and compassion that only one who has been there can have.

Little by little, new changes became routine. Old habits were being replaced by new, healthier ones. I was figuring out who I really was. I felt loved and supported by Erik and my recovery community. I had a strong program attempting to keep myself sober with multiple layers of people and other measures of accountability in place. It started to feel better and the desire to drink began to dissipate. Recovery, in those first few months, was honestly a full time job for me. I drove from counselor appointments to meetings, to my sponsor to the addiction doctor for my shots, back and forth, all over the metro. And as much as I wanted to be filling my time with my family and work, I know it was the right thing and that I had nothing else to focus on but myself for a while. If it sounds selfish, that is because it is. Alcoholism is selfish and destructive. Recovery, strangely, is also selfish—at first especially. It has to be. It takes time and commitment, talking about yourself, learning about yourself, self self self! But, the destruction was gone. I was building my life all over again, and I needed to have a really solid foundation in order to be any good to anyone or anything else.

Chapter Sixteen

RE-ESTABLISHING RELATIONSHIPS WITH MY KIDS

I had lost the trust of my children, their father, their counselor, and their guardian. The well-being of those beautiful kids was first and foremost in the minds of many, including myself. Jim, my ex-husband, the therapist and the guardian all encouraged reunification but set strict parameters for safety.

The first challenge was reunification therapy, with their therapist Jonathan, the kids, and myself. We discussed their fears, how I had hurt them, and tried to figure out if they were ready and willing to have me back in their lives. They wanted to try, but they wanted it to be safe. They were both scared of riding in a car with me, and were relieved to know that I had the ignition interlock again. They were afraid to be alone with me at first, which stung, but I understood. Supervised parenting time was going to be the only way to go about this.

I was able to hire the same woman who had supervised me at my worst the previous fall. She would take me on because I had the ignition interlock, and would only allow a visit to take place once I had blown a 0.00 into my machine. She also could ask me at any moment to do it again. She admitted later that she had been quite nervous about trying again with me, because she had never before been part of such an addiction crisis. She charged thirty dollars per hour, for which I utilized retirement funds to bankroll. She told me she was shocked at how much better I looked—in fact she barely recognized me.

As annoying as it could be to have someone looking over my shoulder, I was very appreciative of her services. Without her, I wouldn't have been able to see the kids. We started slowly, a couple of hours two to three times a week. The visits went well. Tammy and I became friends as time passed. I got more comfortable with having her there. Sometimes we would go somewhere, take the kids out to eat or to an indoor play gym. Sometimes, we stayed at home and played. She was not intrusive, but she was cautious and observant. She was kind. But at all times, her main priority was the kids.

The children began to show signs of being more comfortable again with me. We had some fun. We played games, watched TV, ate together, worked on homework, normal mundane things that were so blissfully awesome to me. I had taken them for granted and was no longer doing that. I would find myself in tears at the smallest achievement or hug. It was clear that trust was going to take a long time to rebuild, especially with my son Tate. My daughter had really missed me and was much quicker to forgive and show her love.

After a couple of months, Erik was allowed to take part in some of the visits so that the kids, the supervisor, and the guardian, could meet him. He was great with them, and they seemed to like him. Tate and Erik would watch sports and talk football. Olivia and Erik joked around a lot and were silly together. Erik's children, Nick and Evelyn, came to stay with us from Pennsylvania a couple of times. The four kids got along quite well.

The guardian and parenting time supervisor were happy with the progress, and about the time I was seven months sober, were ready to try a weekend with overnights. They asked that it be with another trusted adult, and this was my father. Dad agreed to come down and stay the weekend and report to the supervisor any concerns. He talked with her ahead of time regarding the rules. He took the role seriously because of the kids. He wasn't ready to forgive and forget with me, but if I was going to be with my kids, he wanted to make sure it was done safely.

It went well. We had all four kids that weekend. We went to the Mall of America. We ate great food. We watched movies and played games and overall had a terrific time. The guardian and supervisor, as well as my ex-husband, were confident that I could begin unsupervised parenting as long as I kept the ignition interlock in the car and made sure my son had his cell phone charged and ready if he needed anything. Slowly, things advanced to 50/50 parenting time. My relationship with the kids became so real and true. We were able to talk more freely. I was so grateful. I still am.

In the years since I got sober, I have since fully gained back the trust I lost with both Tate and Olivia. They are proud of me. They have confidence in my recovery. The ignition interlock has long since been removed. They no longer sniff my drinks or seem the slightest bit concerned that I will return to drinking. Because I fell on my face in such spectacular fashion, I really have no leg to stand on regarding judging them for any "misdeeds." I am happy for this, because I know my previous self would have aimed for perfection in my children as a reflection on me. I have become honest and have perspective and humility. I had no idea how valuable those recovery skills would become in parenting. The kids can, and do, tell me anything. They have seen what addiction can do, and have no interest in drugs or alcohol. They know they are at a disadvantage because both of their parents are alcoholics, so they have a very healthy fear of it. They have seen that one can make monumental mistakes and still turn it around and become a better person. That can't be taught—it has to be lived, and they have lived it.

I am not happy that I was neglectful and took them for granted and risked their safety, quite the opposite, in fact. I remain guilt ridden about that. Many other things I have been able to let go—but that one sticks. It is a great motivator in maintaining my sobriety. "We will not regret the past (so I don't sit and stew in it) nor wish to shut the door on it (I can NEVER forget what alcohol did to me!!)." But I am grateful that because of my alcoholism and recovery, my relationship with the children is much better than it would have been even had I been able to just control my drinking. I am present. I am not numb. I am here for them in every way. I am far from perfect so how could I expect perfection from them? I am much more patient and forgiving and do not sweat the small stuff like I did before recovery. I am a good person and a good mother. I was not either of those things in active addiction.

I enjoy the small things. Attending a choir concert one of the kids is involved in brings me to joyful tears. Watching my son get his drivers' license was awesome. My daughter has her first boyfriend. Homecoming. Grades. Boy scouts. Tennis. Swimming. Being able to drive them wherever, whenever. Them knowing they can rely on me; them asking me for advice. Our home is a hub of teenage activity, a place where their friends feel comfortable. There are adolescent challenges, sibling bickering and messy rooms. I love it all, every minute. I had it all before and hadn't appreciated any of it. I will not be making that mistake again.

Chapter Seventeen

RETURNING TO WORK

My retirement funds were dwindling. Erik's work as a car salesman was not enough to meet our financial needs. It turned out that his equine business was in shambles and he was unable to find any common ground with his co-owners. I taught more piano lessons. We continued to rely on food assistance. I needed to work. I had a Masters degree; I should be employable in some fashion, even if it wasn't as a PA right away.

When I had eight months of documented sobriety under my belt, I petitioned for reinstatement of my PA license. I met with the Board of Medical Practice in Minneapolis. Others cautioned me to hire an attorney to accompany me. I did not have the funds for that, and I had no intention of lying or trying to get away with anything, so I went alone.

In a boardroom full of a dozen high ranking officials—MD's, lawyers, professionals of many types—I pleaded my case. The board members were kind, I was nervous. I prayed and meditated on my drive there, and in the waiting room ahead of the meeting, to just be honest and be myself. They asked me many questions about my past, my present, my recovery, why this time was different, and why they should consider reinstating me. They asked of my experience with HPSP and if I would be willing to be monitored again.

Through it all, I was honest. HPSP had been nothing but supportive—I had screwed up my involvement with them all on my own and held no resentments towards them. If they would take me on again, I would welcome it. I talked of my children, and renewing relationships with them and other family members. We discussed trust, and how I was working very hard to gain back their trust and that I was doing everything in my power to stay sober and never break that trust again. I told them that I missed my work, I loved being a PA, and that I felt I had a new compassion and empathy that was lacking before. I told them that I wanted to be a PA again, but that I understood if that was not possible. I told them I was willing to go to any lengths to stay sober.

They made it clear that their job is to protect the public. They also stated that they want and need qualified, experienced, sober medical providers in the state of Minnesota. I was asked to leave the room while they deliberated. Praying and trying to meditate during a very long fifteen minutes really didn't ease my mind, but I ended my prayers with "thy will, not mine." I got my license back.

Obviously, it was a restricted license. I was to immediately be enrolled in HPSP for monitoring. Any potential position I would take as a PA would require Board approval and had to be a large multiple provider facility. I was limited to twenty-four hours per week direct patient care, with no call. Assigned to me was a member of the Board, my direct contact and someone with whom I was required to meet quarterly. This, along with continued counseling, medication treatment, meetings, work site monitor reports, reports from my sponsor, and drug and alcohol monitoring indefinitely.

I was elated that I was being given a second chance. Potential employers, however, not so much. Nobody really wants to hire a PA who was recently drunk out of her mind, in rehab, on HPSP, with the ability to work a max of twenty-four hours a week and no ability to cover call. So began the job search.

After a month of running into brick walls because of the restrictions, I began to look outside of clinical medicine. Quality assurance, electronic medical record specialist, prior authorizations for insurance companies—I interviewed for all but nothing was working out. A medical publishing company, Elsevier, was looking for clinical editors. What in the hell is a clinical editor? It turns out it is a trained clinician (RN, PA, MD) who writes articles and patient education and medical textbooks. Writes and edits for accuracy. A clinical editor continually follows current medical guidelines and adjusts literature accordingly. Active or restricted or no license—didn't matter. They wanted the degree and the experience. I took the job. It paid about half of what I had been paid as a full time PA, but it was still nothing to sneeze at. I was so grateful to work and get my fingers back in medicine, even if I wasn't seeing patients. A biweekly paycheck to put in my overdrawn account was such a relief.

The hours were full time, Monday-Friday 8-5. I was still able to fully commit to my recovery program, simply adjusting some times of meetings with my sponsor and choosing evening meetings to attend rather than daytime meetings. I found a facility near work where I could go for my observed urine collections on the days my color was called. The ignition interlock remained in the car. The safeguards were all in place, I just had to make some adjustments. It felt so good to be productive. To be putting out good work that was medically focused. To be working with a team of other educated people trying to create excellent literature.

Erik continued to work at the car dealership. We saw his kids periodically. They spent quite a bit of the summer with us. My kids were with us about half the time. Just four months after having met Erik at rehab, he proposed. He walked into the kitchen where I was washing dishes, handed me a box with a ring in it. I was surprised; he said "You know we're going to do it, so why not now?"

The stark contrast between my first proposal at Disneyworld with fireworks and this one in the kitchen with my dishwater hands was not lost on me. It made me feel good, the lack of show, the lack of grandeur. I loved him. He loved me. He accepted me, flaws and all. He didn't care what anyone else thought. We were in recovery together. We went to meetings together. We were making a life with our children. Marriage, though I had vowed never to get married again, seemed a logical next step. I said yes.

CᴓᴑChapter Eighteenᴓᴑᴐ

MARRIAGE #2

E rik and I had such a lovely relationship. It was so comfortable. He understood me and my flaws, accepted me for who I was, supported me unconditionally. He helped soothe me when I felt lonely for my children or when I struggled because repairing relationships with my family was a slow process. He encouraged me to continue working my program, but didn't try to run it for me. He supported my efforts towards gaining back the trust of my parents and sister. Because of his alcoholism, as well as some significant family dysfunction, he and his parents and only sister were not speaking. Erik's children lived in Pennsylvania most of the time, but did come to see us about four times a year, sometimes for several weeks at a time. So he understood the pain that comes along with broken relationships and helped me to be patient yet persistent. He didn't want me to feel the same loss he had with his family.

We went to a lot of meetings together at first. I moved forward with my sponsor. Erik floated around a bit, never quite finding a sponsor that worked for him. He dwelled on the past, particularly his relationships with his parents and sister. He could not seem to make any headway in repairing things, yet perseverated on those issues as well as his lost business. He was often stuck in a rut of not knowing what to do with his life without that. I listened, encouraged, supported. I told him of the things that were helping with my recovery, but he didn't feel those things would benefit him. He became increasingly dissatisfied with his work as a car salesman. I was set to begin my new job at the medical publishing company the week following our wedding and we discussed that if he was still that unhappy once I started work, he would look for something different.

We planned a small wedding on a yacht. I paid for it with the remaining money from my retirement accounts. The wedding day fell on my nine-month sobriety anniversary. There were about twenty-five people there to celebrate with us, including my sister and her family as well as my parents, a cousin and his wife, and my aunt and uncle. My sponsor Judy, my friends Tami, Patty, Jeanne, Lauren, and Maureen attended. Our sons, Nick and Tate, wore rented tuxedos along with Erik. Our girls, Olivia and Evelyn, wore cream colored satin gowns that matched mine. When we said our vows, we also said vows to our new stepchildren. I had chosen all of the verses and words, including the serenity prayer. It was such a moving and personal ceremony and evening. Besides Erik's children, he had invited his parents and sister, who had declined. He had invited his best friend from out East who had also declined. Erik had no one there other than his children. My mother said that she had enough love to act as both of our mothers that day, which meant a great deal to Erik.

Erik had begun a spiritual relapse, as clear in hindsight by the lack of enthusiasm for recovery, general dissatisfaction with life and work, living in the past, and feeling unimportant. I believe that once I had solid footing and found an entire support network in recovery, he felt less needed, less important, and like I didn't need his help anymore. I think he was feeling very useless and depressed. Shortly before our wedding, I noticed that he seemed more energetic. His lazy eye which usually only showed up when he was extremely tired, began to appear more frequently. He was chewing gum a lot, and when I would go to kiss him, he would cough or do something to deter me. Even when making love, he would turn his head from me and avoid kissing. I knew what was happening in my heart. I knew he had started drinking again. I wanted to be wrong and hoped I was. Finally, I confronted him and he admitted it.

It was like the floor fell out beneath me. What happened to our team? What happened to being in this sobriety thing together? I felt so scared, sad, and betrayed.

I still married him.

I felt like, together, we could get him to stop and be happy. I felt that, as an alcoholic myself, I needed to be supportive and helpful, and not abandon him in his time of need. He put on a good show for a bit, going to more meetings, talking more with me. He refused to get a new sponsor, though, and did not want to see a counselor or psychiatrist. He said he couldn't talk to those people; he could only talk to me. I was his "only." It was draining, but I tried my hardest. I quickly became the best damned enabler who ever lived. I wanted him to stop drinking. I wanted him to be happy. I knew if I left him, he would deteriorate and be so incredibly lonely that I didn't know if he would survive. I loved him so much, he had helped me so much and I felt that I owed him this support. I felt certain that if it was me that had relapsed, he would stand by me.

The day after the wedding, Erik quit his job at the car dealership. He apparently just stopped going, I was later told by his previous boss. He left all his personal effects there, never returning to get his pictures, or papers, or anything. Just never went back. Meanwhile, I started my new, full time job at the publishing company. We had a great deal of debt—treatment center bills, Erik's old cell phone and electric bills. A credit card that was maxed out I could no longer pay. We got behind in our rent payments and car payments. I was providing medical and dental insurance through my work to all of us, including his kids in Pennsylvania. We had to pay 750 dollars a month to his ex-wife for child support. My ex-husband sued me for some double child support payments he had made, and he won, leaving me with more debt from both him and the lawyer I had hired to represent me. I was making decent money, but Erik was making none, and he was spending more and more on alcohol. He took a position as the assistant football coach at the local high school. He told them he didn't need to be paid! I was shocked and told him we really needed the money, but he needed to feel better about himself and by acting as if he didn't need money to the head coach, I guess that made him feel good.

I tried explaining to him, in a kind way, that our bills were mounting and that I was feeling incredibly stressed. I took on more piano students to try to help. He continued to work—for free—for the football team and go to the bars. He didn't bring any alcohol into the house at first, but bars are expensive. I didn't know what to do. I tried nagging, I cried, I got angry, but he didn't seem to understand. I couldn't believe that I was now on this side of the disease of alcoholism. It certainly provided a whole lot of clarity as to what I had put my parents, sister, and children through. I was working, cooking, cleaning, shopping, taking care of the kids, paying for Nick and Evelyn's flights here, entertaining them while they were here and Erik was drunk or passed out, paying for their child support, AND I WAS TRYING TO STAY SOBER! I kept going to meetings; I was honest with my sponsor about the situation. She never told me what to do, but was hopeful for him and helped me stay on task with my own recovery.

Finally, I told him he absolutely needed to get a paying job. He took one through a temp agency working in a manufacturing plant. He cut pieces of metal to a specific length—all day. It was mind numbing for him. He hated it. He drank more. He got a corneal abrasion a couple weeks in from a piece of hot metal, and never went back.

Finding him sobbing on the couch one evening when I returned from work, he asked me to take him somewhere. I took him to Fairview, the very first place I had gone for detox—you know, the one where I tried to break out with a bobby pin? Yeah, that one. It felt awful weird to be going through the whole thing but as the spouse, not the addict. Those three days where he was in detox were so relaxing for me. I was able to rest, sleep, not worry that my bedmate was going to die in the night. He seemed committed to staying sober and was so very apologetic and sad, depressed, hopeless. I couldn't abandon him. I needed to keep trying to help. I knew what a great man he was, deep inside.

For a while, he would work bits of the program and white-knuckle sobriety. Then he would relapse. He would feel worse and each relapse was more devastating physically, emotionally, and financially than the last. He tried Antabuse, but drank right through that. He did not work for many months. I kept robbing Peter to pay Paul to somehow keep the landlord and the creditors off my back, but I was drowning in debt and feeling trapped. On and on this went. He always had food to eat, a roof over his head, a car to drive, and money to buy booze. Enable much, Karla? I was in survival mode—just working my ass off at work and at home to try to keep our lives afloat. He was in alcoholic survival mode—just figuring out how to keep drinking and sleeping every day away so he didn't have to actually feel anything. At some point I told him he could not go to the bars anymore, it was too expensive. He then started bringing the alcohol into the house. I felt it was a lesser evil—at least he was not out driving around and he wasn't spending quite as much money on booze. Though, he drank a LOT. Like thirty beers a day and sometimes some scotch mixed in. (And that is only the booze I knew about—I am sure it was much more that was hidden.)

Many people asked how I could do that. How could I have alcohol in my house and be faced with it every day? It was pretty simple, actually. I was repulsed by the smell and the behavior and the laziness and I hated the disease of alcoholism even more than I had previously. There was one moment, when I accidentally discovered a bottle of Smirnoff in the laundry room. I was frustrated and angry; I was defeated and felt trapped. I looked at that bottle. I opened it. I took a long smell. I even tipped the bottle up toward my lips. But, I played the tape forward. I realized what would happen, what I would lose, if I took that first sip. So, I didn't and I have rarely been tempted since.

On and on this went. He was in and out of detox a handful of times, each time I was hopeful, but each time he didn't truly change anything. Our financial state worsened, yet he refused to see that it was a serious problem. We got evicted because we were four months behind in our rent payments. I still had decent enough credit to buy a small house, with a down payment provided by my parents. I downsized my car from a suburban to a small SUV. He began to sell Aflac insurance for a while, but that required overnight trips out of town often. With that came hotel rooms and dinners out and booze. The money was flying out of the account much faster than he could even conceive of making back. Yet he refused to see it this way, refused to acknowledge how bad it was. He would not provide me with receipts that I could at least keep tallied for tax breaks. I finally told him his working for Aflac was costing us more than it was providing, so he happily quit.

I began to realize that I shouldn't and couldn't keep on like this. I gave him an ultimatum—sobriety or divorce. He got a new sponsor, Bob. He came up with a contract to stay sober and consequences if he didn't. He blew right through that contract and started drinking again. I took away his debit card at different times. He would scrounge through drawers for change and still go buy alcohol. He was so addicted that we both knew he could not just stop cold turkey. He used that to his advantage and I would give him his card back. Finally, I had enough. We set a move out date for him. I was so angry and felt so used and betrayed, drained emotionally and financially. I just wanted him gone. I felt that I had made a big mistake in marrying him, and that my counselor back in Florida had been absolutely correct in warning me against this. But, what was done was done. I don't even recall where he was planning to go—I think a sober house. His kids were with us at the time as it was summertime, so we agreed that once they went back to Pennsylvania, he would move out. In fact, every time his kids came to visit, for some reason his drinking escalated exponentially. I began to be able to predict it. But I wanted to see my stepchildren, and I knew they should see their dad, so I continued to pay for their plane tickets, and pick them up at the airport, attempt to entertain them while they were here while their dad often was unavailable, and passed out in bed. It was such a vicious cycle. I was done. He was going to move out in two weeks.

Slicing up meat and cheese one night for everyone, I had this overwhelming sense of nausea and dizziness. I thought I might faint. I ended up dropping to the kitchen floor and just sitting there for a few minutes before it passed. Got up, smelled the meat, nauseated again. What in the world?

Oh my God. I had felt this way before, when I was pregnant. But I was forty-one-years old, taking birth control pills faithfully every night, had a light period a couple weeks previously, and could recall only one time in the past six weeks that Erik and I had been intimate. Maybe it was early menopause. Or maybe I was getting the flu. The stick read "pregnant" twice, in the public restroom at my work the following day. A startled woman in the next stall asked me if I was alright after I screamed "Oh My God."

Well, this was going to complicate things. Erik was drinking; I had become angry and irritated, as well as resentful. I felt spent both emotionally and financially. But, I wanted this baby. I was healthy and sober, and had always wanted another child. This was a miracle to me, and I was ready to raise the baby all by myself.

Lying in bed that night next to Erik, having just had another heated discussion about his drinking and his moving out, I realized I needed to tell him. I said "Erik?" He said "Karla?" I said "I'm pregnant." He said "what? how?" and then he asked "is it mine"? Talk about making a bad situation worse. I was very upset, obviously, and assured him that it was indeed his, that I had not now or ever cheated on him, and that I wanted this baby. He said "so do I." Then he quickly reasoned that he should not be moving out into sober living or a halfway house, he needed to step it up and be there for me and the baby.

He agreed to try another round at detox, this time it was a public crappy detox in Hastings, MN, where typically they send inmates to detox before going back to jail. We couldn't afford anything else and still owed money to Fairview from his last detox. He cried and drank all the way to detox, apologizing, making promises, and I dropped him off in a dark, frightening back stairway where the nurse took him and told me I couldn't go in. I felt awful leaving him there, but knew I had to. Another blissful three days of peace and serenity at home with my teenagers provided respite to me.

He tried to stay sober once out, but simply couldn't. He again didn't want counseling or to see a doctor. He did not buy into the 12 steps anymore and refused that. He would not call his old sponsor. He just tried, again, to white knuckle it. But before too many days, I would see his eyes appear crossed, and the jovial demeanor returned, quickly followed by the crash and burn. He was not working. Meanwhile, I went to OB appointments (twice weekly ultrasounds because I was considered a high risk "advanced maternal age" patient and the baby had a bout of tachycardia), continued to work full time, and had begun my quest toward removing the work hours and call restrictions set upon me by the Board of Medical Practice, because I wanted professionally and needed financially to return to clinical practice if I was ever going to get my head above water and be able to support the new baby.

Despite his drinking, it was clear Erik was also excited about the baby. He wanted to do this, and I could hear in his words and see in his face how badly he wanted to do it right—to do it sober. But the drink kept winning. It was taking him down. And it was trying to take me down with it. Alcohol was still ruining my life, but I wasn't even getting to get drunk.

I continued to be diligent about my meetings and seeing my sponsor, along with seeing my counselor and addiction specialist. Insurance stopped covering the Vivitrol shots after about a year, so I stopped getting them because I couldn't afford $1,600 dollars a month. Thankfully, no cravings returned. I am unsure if it actually ever helped me other than through a placebo effect, but I am glad I had it on board for as long as I did. My urine monitoring continued, and months under my belt of proven sobriety kept adding up. After a year of sobriety, the kids and my ex agreed that I no longer needed the ignition interlock, so that was removed, taking with it an eighty-nine dollar per month payment, for which I was grateful.

I tried to keep juggling money around and putting off creditors. We got a month behind in our house payment. Then we got behind in the car payments. Ultimately, Erik's car was repossessed. He needed a car, because he was now actively searching for a new job to try to help support us. So, I leased a car, in my name because he had no credit or income. In a few months, the new car was also repossessed, though I was able to pay an exorbitant amount of money in a hurry to get it back. I now had a mortgage and two cars in my name, as well as a credit card balance of 25K—none of which I could pay on time. My credit had tanked. There was the ongoing $750 dollars a month child support along with the electric, cable and cell phone bills; groceries gasoline, car insurance. We still owed our old landlord $12,000 dollars, and he served us with a civil lawsuit. We settled on a payment plan, 500 dollars a month. I was so stressed about money. I talked to Erik about it all of the time. I printed out bank statements, tallied up the costs of alcohol, tallied up the amount of cash he pulled out every month, showed him a budget, even attempted to hire a credit expert to help us with a budget. Nothing changed. He even ended up hanging up on the credit expert because he was certain their services were a scam. The only thing I knew how to do to get us out of this mess was to make more money.

C♪Chapter Nineteen♫⌒

RETURN TO CLINICAL MEDICINE

Given that I had lost my national board certification after surrendering my Minnesota PA license, I needed to start from scratch and take boards all over again in an attempt to recertify. Taking boards is never an easy task, but it certainly went smoother than I expected it would. I studied hard, did practice exams, and retained information much better than I had in the past—spoiler alert—drinking makes it hard to learn and remember anything! I passed the boards on the first try. So, I had my board certification back and my Minnesota license, though it was restricted.

I petitioned at one year of sobriety to have the hours and call restrictions lifted. Meeting with the board, we discussed my program, and the fact that I had been working full time, albeit not in clinical medicine, without relapsing. Pleading that it was going to prove difficult to find a position working just twenty-four hours a week without call that would include benefits that I needed for my family, I stressed that I wouldn't be able to find a job. The board agreed, the hours and call restrictions were lifted. The "restricted" black mark remained on my license however, until my HPSP monitoring was complete.

Eventually, I would need to reapply for my DEA license which I had also lost. Without it, I wouldn't be employable because I wouldn't be able to prescribe medications. Cost prohibited me from doing that until I could find PA employment that would cover the cost, so I had no choice but to wait. There was not even room on one of my credit cards for the $731 dollar price tag for a new DEA license.

About six months into my position in medical publishing, and no longer having the constraints of limited hours and no call attached to my license, I began to search in earnest for a clinical PA position. I was unsure of how much to disclose to potential employers. Do I tell them I am in recovery and being monitored by HPSP? Do I wait until I have an offer and then tell them? If they won't interview me because of my history of alcoholism, isn't that discrimination? All of these questions and so many more flooded my brain and I was anxious and overwhelmed at times. Relying heavily on Step Three (thy will, not mine), as well as the near constant advice and support from my sponsor and other friends in recovery got me through each day without drinking.

During my first interview, I did not disclose my alcoholism. I did not tell them my license was restricted or that I was involved in HPSP. The interview went great, and

I was offered a job which would pay $40,000 more annually than I was making in publishing. I accepted the job. Upon completing paperwork to become credentialed by insurance companies, I disclosed my situation. The CEO personally called me to rescind the offer and told me that it wasn't even the drinking past or monitoring that upset him, but that I hadn't disclosed it to him during the interview process. I was crushed. It was a huge milestone for me, however, in that I learned once again that honesty is the best policy. I couldn't let my fears get in the way of doing what was right, and that meant being honest. I was crushed, but I did not drink.

I went with the "whole truth, nothing but the truth, so help me God" attitude to my next interview. This would be a four day per week position at a VA outpatient clinic. Given so many veterans struggle with active addiction, or are in recovery, this appealed to me greatly. I had worked at a VA for a few months when I had first graduated PA school and left it only because I wanted to move closer to my family. I was honest from the first meeting. I disclosed my alcoholism, monitoring, restricted license, the whole thing. The panel of interviewers expressed gratitude that I had been upfront, and assured me that they felt my being in recovery could only be beneficial within the VA system. They wanted me. I wanted the job. The pay and benefits were excellent, and included a sign on bonus, which I badly needed for the down payment on the house I was hoping to buy.

To be sure that everyone was on board with hiring me despite my history, I was asked to go and meet with the Chief Medical Officer of the VA hospital in Minneapolis. He was fantastic! We discussed medicine and recovery, children and goals. He agreed with the decision to hire me. I accepted the offer immediately, which was also right about the time we had received the eviction notice from our previous landlord. I then put an offer in on the small new house, which was accepted, and banked on that 10K sign on bonus being available.

A start date was set, and I was so excited. We were within a couple weeks of closing on the house. I felt like I was finally going to be able to repair some of the financial damage in my life and be able to start helping patients again, doing what I love. Three days later, a human resources representative called me and rescinded the offer. She told me that the VA will not hire any medical providers with restricted licenses, even if the restriction is simply that they are being monitored through HPSP. I was so sad. I pleaded with her, and explained that I had disclosed this to EVERYONE during the application and interview process, and that it never should have gone this far. She apologized and empathized, but it was their policy—at the federal level. She told me that sometimes the local offices are unaware of this policy. I called the medical director and the physicians who I had first met with. They were all upset and frustrated. They were going to have to start from scratch to fill the position, and none of them had been aware that the VA had that policy. I even wrote a letter to the medical director of the VA at the federal level in Washington DC. Apparently, a federal law is rather difficult to change, and I never heard back from them. I did, however, hear back from the chief medical officer in Minneapolis, asking how long my license was going to be restricted. With another two years on HPSP ahead of me, neither I nor they could wait.

I remember calling my parents. I felt so defeated. Dad was very concerned that this disappointment would drive me to drink. It didn't. I worked my program and kept working in my publishing job while continually scanning online job opportunities. My parents graciously loaned me the 10K that I needed for the house down payment. I am sure they did this more for the kids than for me or certainly Erik, but it was such a blessing nonetheless. Now I could add yet another person or entity to whom I owed money to my long list of debts. The fear of financial collapse was very real.

PrairieCare provides mental health services to kids and adults, outpatient, partial inpatient and inpatient. They had advertised for a PA in their brand new adolescent inpatient hospital. The position would involve caring for the medical issues the kids had while inpatient. If they had asthma or diabetes, the PA would manage that. If they got hurt or sick while they were inpatient, the PA would manage that. Every child admitted needed an admission physical examination which was also part of the job. These kids had significant mental health issues, often along with suicidal thoughts or attempts, cutting or other self- injury and substance abuse. With a full team of psychiatrists, psychologists, therapists, social workers, case managers, spiritual advisors, nurses, and psychiatric technicians to work with the patients as well, the job description was quite clear—the medical consultant (the PA position's formal title) would not manage the patient's mental health conditions, just the physical issues. The position appealed to me greatly and I felt I could make a real difference for the patients because I understood those dark thoughts and reliance on substances. I understood what it felt like to be locked up in some facility where things were out of my control. I understood the hopelessness and the feeling that one had destroyed their life beyond repair. I wanted to help these kids and give back however I could. I applied immediately.

After being called in for an interview, I spent a lot of time praying and talking to my sponsor and other recovery friends about how to handle the interview. I ultimately decided that I would disclose that I was an alcoholic, in recovery for eighteen months, monitored by HPSP, and tell them that I would be happy to divulge any information regarding this upon request—but that I would not just spend ten minutes talking about and dwelling on my alcoholism history, unless they wanted me to. They did not.

They nodded and appreciated my candor, had only a few questions regarding that, and we moved on to the details of the position. The interview went very well. They called me in for a second interview, in which I would also meet my potential supervising physician and the Chief Medical Officer, to make sure that they were both comfortable with me and my history. Sitting across from who would become my supervising physician, a sweet woman perhaps twenty-years older than me with near crippling rheumatoid arthritis, she leaned forward in her chair and said "I think this would only be an asset to our company." Everyone agreed! I would later come to find out that three of the people sitting at that interview table were in long-term recovery and that the facility was very recovery supportive.

I was offered the job formally a few days later. Full benefits, and a pay increase of 40K annually from what I was earning in publishing. Thank the Lord! I accepted the position, with a start date in just two weeks. I was asked to write letters of explanation to be provided to third party payers like Blue Cross and Medicare, and there were no hold ups in credentialing. I disclosed that I was pregnant, and that was not a concern. There were four of us medical consultants with my arrival, and juggling coverage was up to us which was awesome. No need for administration to get involved, we figured it out amongst ourselves. I started with such hope and fervor, I loved the job immediately, had great rapport with the kids. I believe I will work with PrairieCare as long as they will have me, or until retirement, whichever comes first. I love this job! I am able to do Twelve-Step work at work. I have so much more empathy and compassion for my patients than I had before. I do a very good job, I am efficient, and my memory is sharper than it was when I was in my twenties, all because I no longer drink.

Erik, however, continued to struggle. He went back to detox another time during my pregnancy and found a job working for Comcast, selling their services to businesses. It paid 40K annually, and it kept him busy so he could spend less money and time on drinking. But, he still drank every day on the way home from work and all evening until he passed out. But, he was trying. He wasn't working a program, had pretty much cut out anything recovery related from his life and rarely talked to his sponsor, Bob, mainly because he felt embarrassed that he was still drinking.

We spent Christmas that year up at my parent's home. My mother rented out a four bedroom suite at the local motel so that my family (all six of us, as Nick and Ev were with us), and my sister's family could stay there as my parents' home is not large enough for everyone to sleep in. Erik and Nick drove separately. When they arrived, they had both been drinking—Nick was only seventeen at the time. Erik, especially, was loud and obnoxious when he arrived. My father does not handle others being that way, or when people interrupt and are rude. He made some comment to Erik to tone it down, and before I knew it, Erik and Nick left. They drove back the five-hour drive the next morning, leaving me and the three other kids at my parents. Our family picture that year makes me sad—I am quite pregnant, and Erik and Nick are missing from the picture, all because of alcohol. Once again, alcohol was managing to ruin my life. I felt so trapped, though, but I felt somewhat hopeful because at least now I had a better paying job and Erik was making SOME money rather than just spending.

After Nick and Evelyn flew home following the holidays, Erik's drinking went rapidly downhill. He started calling in sick for work. He then broke his ankle. A drunk and injured Erik was no fun. He had surgery. I had to take him to and from these appointments, go to my own OB appointments, get Tate and Olivia to and from their activities, work full time, continue to pay bills and do the shopping and on and on—PLUS care for a whiny, demanding, drunk (and high on oxycodone) husband. It was awful. He learned to drive with his boot so he could buy more alcohol. He always found a way to get the booze, but couldn't find a way to help me around the house or do anything that wasn't self-serving. It was such a dose of reality for me, once again reminding me of what I had previously put my family through during my drinking days. It seemed there was no saving him. During this time, I went into premature labor and had to be hospitalized for two days to stop it. He and the kids came to visit me, and he smelled of booze and limped around clumsily on his crutches and I was really upset because he had driven the kids that way. I asked him not to bring the kids again. I couldn't rely on my ex-husband at that time, either, because he had returned to his alcoholic ways as well. The stress was indescribable.

About two weeks before my due date, Erik asked to go to rehab. We contacted Hazelden and they would take him. I had to pay a large sum upfront and then insurance would cover the rest. I took him up there for his intake. He drank and sobbed the whole drive. He was so apologetic, he said all of the right things, and he wanted to get straight before the baby came. He seemed ready and committed and I was so grateful. Breathing out many sighs of relief on my way home, alone, that evening, I felt a sense of peace and serenity that had been lacking for quite some time.

I went to visit him twice a week during the facility visiting hours. I continued to attend my twice weekly ultrasounds, work full time, and take care of my two teenagers. Evelyn and Nick had been planning to come for the birth, which was scheduled for March 16th (due to my age, a planned induction at thirty-nine weeks was standard.) I knew I could not add them to my list of things to handle, so I contacted Erik's sister who took care of notifying their mother and cancelling the trip. It was the first and only time I have ever spoken to her. It was evident in her voice and her words that she was fed up with him and would only take my call because of the kids. She wished me well, though, and felt awful for the situation. Nick called as well, and asked what I was going to do. I told him honestly I did not know, but at that moment all I could focus on was getting safely through the delivery. Evelyn called too, though I could barely understand her because she was sobbing. She so wanted to meet the new baby and be there for the birth, but it simply wasn't possible. I felt terrible about that.

Erik called my parents to tell them of his situation. He cried to them and apologized and asked them to come be with me. So they did, and for that I am eternally grateful. They managed my house and took care of Tate and Olivia. Mom accompanied me to some of my ultrasounds. We had a lovely time. It was so peaceful and normal and boring, which was just fine with me! Of course, being forty-two years old and needing my parents to come "save the day"—again—was a bit deflating. My counselor helped me to simply be grateful and not dwell on any guilt or shame associated with the situation. I tried, and succeeded for the most part, but there were certainly times where I felt a sense of self-pity.

Sawyer

With the induction date rapidly approaching, Erik was able to secure a pass to have his sponsor bring him to and from the hospital the day of delivery. He had to be back to Hazelden by 10 P.M. though. My mother and I arrived at the hospital at 7:30 in the morning as scheduled. My father stayed behind to drive Tate and Olivia to and from school and care for them afterwards. I was clear with the nurses and physicians that I wanted no mood altering medications—no Demerol, no Fentanyl in my epidural, just lidocaine. The anesthesiologist tried to talk me out of that, but I was firm. My HPSP case worker was aware of the impending delivery and gave me a three day window to not worry about providing any UA's, and told me to send her a discharge summary which would cover me if I tested positive for anything that they had administered during birth. But I didn't want to risk my sobriety, and continued to refuse any narcotics.

Erik and his sponsor Bob arrived mid-morning. Bob wandered around the hospital, left for a while here and there to do some work, and Erik mainly slept on the little couch in the room. My mother left for a bit to go get Olivia who wanted to be present for the birth. They arrived, but didn't stay long as Olivia started feeling very ill. Turns out she had Influenza A. Labor was fairly easy. The lidocaine epidural was moderately effective until the last stages. At 7 P.M. I was only at four centimeters. Everyone was watching the clock because Erik had to leave at 9:00 P.M. My previous births I had progressed rapidly from four to ten centimeters and this birth was no different. Bob left to go to the cafeteria to get some sodas. By the time he returned, I had progressed to ten centimeters and the staff were rushing around to find a doctor, ANY doctor, to catch this baby. At 7:30 P.M., little Sawyer David was born weighing in at six pounds eleven ounces, nineteen inches long, and perfect in every way. Erik held him, we cried, took some Polaroid pictures that he could bring back to rehab, and Bob had to take him back. I should mention that Bob went far above and beyond to help us; he says it's because it's what he does in the program. I think that is partly true, but also that he is just an incredible guy. He has, to this day, continued to support Erik and me. He is Sawyer's Godfather.

Sawyer and I were moved to a tiny room, very cozy in a corner of the hospital, for we no longer needed the large delivery room which was soon to be required for another delivering mom. I loved the time with my new infant; just him and me. He was a great eater and sleeper immediately. He was so beautiful. They came and took pictures of us—the hospital does that for all the new babies. I spent a couple hundred dollars on those pictures because they turned out great—sort of the Disney package for new Moms, and impossible to resist. The next day, both Sawyer and I had surgery. He a circumcision, me a tubal ligation. As much as I loved this baby, I knew it had been a miracle that he was born healthy without any abnormalities related to my age, and I did not want to risk another pregnancy.

It was kind of sad being wheeled into the operating room without my husband there to support me. My parents were busy running around with Tate and Olivia and managing my house. Erik was in rehab. So, I went in to surgery alone. I still have resentment about that; it's small, but it still is there. I am working on it, though. I had visits from my friends Jeanne and Lisa, my mother, and my son Tate. Shortly after delivery, my sister and her three girls surprised us with a visit to meet the newborn! Olivia was not allowed in the hospital sadly, because of her influenza.

Two days later, my mother arrived to take me and little Sawyer home. Because of the tubal ligation, they wanted to give me Percocet. I declined, and reminded them of my addiction history. I used ibuprofen and that was quite effective. I didn't want to have a fuzzy head and risk relapse. When we got to the parking ramp, the nurse who had wheeled me out got a call from another nurse telling her to wait, she had something for me. The second nurse came flying into the parking ramp to hand me a prescription for Percocet. I said I didn't want it, wouldn't fill it, wouldn't take it. She said "well, I have it right here, you should just take it." I finally had to say, "Look, I am a drunk, and I am in recovery, and I want to stay in recovery, which means no opiates." She finally relented but had a confused look on her face. I have found that even within the medical community, addiction is poorly understood and managed. I hadn't understood it either as a medical professional and recalled in my PA training approximately two hours of the twenty-seven month program being related to addiction. It is frustrating and rather shocking, considering the epidemic of opiate abuse and alcoholism in this country.

Safely home, we settled into a nice routine. My parents were amazing. They cooked and shopped, kept the house in order, and cared for the older kids. Sawyer had jaundice and required the bilirubin lights at home for several days, along with home nurse visits to keep checking his weight and coloring and heel sticks for bilirubin levels. He thrived, got off the lights, and I had enough energy to release my parents to finally get back to their own lives.

Considering I had worked less than a year at PrairieCare, I did not have a great deal of paid time off accrued and I could not afford to take any days off without pay, so I planned to take just six weeks off for maternity leave. My colleagues covered my absence graciously. I searched for a daycare to accept an infant and found a terrific little center near my workplace. I continued to meet with my sponsor and attend meetings. Erik continued with his inpatient treatment, and his counselors recommended he stay longer than the twenty-eight days due to his lengthy history of drinking and recurrent relapses. The older kids did well with school and activities and really enjoyed the baby. During my maternity leave after my parents left, I flew Nick and Evelyn out to meet Sawyer and took them to visit Erik at Hazelden. Nick even attended the family program, which I drove him to and from for three days. Neither of Erik's kids was very hopeful about his recovery, but they sure enjoyed Sawyer. Nick was such a young man during that time—helping with chores and anything I might need, always asking before he went to bed if there was anything else I needed. Evelyn, well with her there, I didn't need to do much at all with the baby. She was in love and she was such a little mommy. It was joyful to watch and be part of it, but it was also sad that Erik was missing out on all of the bonding taking place.

Erik stayed in extended care rehab until mid-May, when Sawyer was about three months old. Coming home, he was great! He worked his program, went to meetings, helped me care for Sawyer, and returned to work at Comcast. Things were good for about two months. Then, his lazy eye began to show. He began to reveal signs that he was drinking again, more demanding, perseverating on ideas and the past, relying on me to manage the household and take care of the kids. I confronted him about it, he admitted it. I asked him to call his sponsor, he wouldn't. I asked him to go to meetings, he refused. My friend Lisa even tried to talk to him about his drinking, but he wasn't going to budge. He lasted a few months at his job and was fired.

Again, the drinking at the bars was too costly. I felt myself sinking again financially. He brought the booze back in, as it was cheaper that way. He agreed to try another rehab, this time it was in Michigan. But three days in, he called stating he couldn't stay there. I had done some research after he had been admitted, and their program was unorthodox and the reviews were horrid. It was, apparently, scientology based and they were administering phenobarbital to their clients in a purple juice cocktail while stripping them of all their other medications. So when he called, I let him come home.

He came home sober and committed to staying that way; he never wanted to return to another rehab like that. He did not return to meetings or work with a sponsor, just tried to go along on willpower, which of course, did not last. Before long, he was back to just as bad, if not worse, than before. Two more detox stays followed. His unemployment benefits ran out. I took a second and then third job covering urgent care shifts while he stayed home and sort of watched Sawyer. His idea of babysitting was Sawyer in the living room watching nickelodeon all day, while Erik sat in bed drinking, watching sports, and dozing. I did not know what to do. The money was flying out of the account. Again I tried taking his credit card, and again he found change and reasons for me to give back the card.

Sometime during all of this, I petitioned to the Minnesota Board of Medical Practice for my unrestricted license, because they had stipulated that I could after three years. My board representative encouraged me to do it because, frankly, I believe he was tired of seeing me every three months and having nothing to discuss because I was maintaining my program. I met in front of the board, AGAIN, and told them that I was very happy in my program and that my unrestricted license was not inhibiting my work in any way, and that I was really only petitioning at the request of my Board representative. I told them I would be happy to have a restricted license and stay on HPSP for the rest of my life, if necessary.

They didn't feel that was necessary. My unrestricted license was granted. And just like that, I was done with HPSP and the monitoring that came along with it. It wasn't even a relief because it had become just a way of life for me, calling in for my color every day, going in whenever needed for UA's. It was going to be nice to stop peeing in front of people, but then again, that wasn't really the case because I had a toddler who followed me everywhere— including into the bathroom!

Erik eventually found work as a paraprofessional at a daycare center. This was the best job for him, because he loved children and he could not drink on the job. He was the classroom assistant, so he did not have to manage the lesson plans or attend parent conferences. He would drink as soon as he got off work, though, until he passed out at night. But, at least he was bringing in a little money, not enough to cover his car and child support and alcohol and cigarettes, but enough that we could get by. We were overdrawn every two weeks, taking out cash to float on with overdraft fees like crazy. We would split up the cash to last us until my payday. His was gone in two days, excuses like gasoline, but I knew the truth. I had to make mine last for milk and diapers and gasoline, and I was working almost all the time. His flight of ideas was back, and he talked of going back to college to become a licensed teacher and coach. I had no idea how we were going to fund that, and also did not believe he could truly do well taking classes in his state of addiction. He then decided to return to the racetrack.

Horse racing had been his life for many years, prior to his moving to Minnesota. He bullied and badgered his way into his dream job at Canterbury Park, about an hour from home. It was truly an excellent job, Racehorse Ownership Ambassador. They were going to pay him $5000 a month. I was thrilled because we needed the money and I hoped it would make him happy. But I felt a great deal of fear as well because drinking and the racetrack go hand in hand. I was concerned that he would drink all day long, drive home, continue drinking, and get worse. I saw the credit card bills; he was spending money left and right, buying drinks for "clients," never submitting receipts to his boss for reimbursement, over tipping, acting like big shot Erik.

I kept working, still managed to go to at least one meeting a week and see my sponsor weekly. I continued to work with my own sponsees and went to the jail once a month or so. My family and friends in and out of the program were beginning to encourage me to kick him out. I threatened him with that, and he threatened me with "squatter's rights," and that I would have to formally evict him, and that he would fight for Sawyer. It was one thing to have him in my house watching Sawyer, where I knew the teenagers were also there in the event of an emergency. It was a completely different idea to consider that if we separated, he may have time with Sawyer completely unsupervised. That scared me into paralysis and indecision. So, I kept going along with working like a dog, trying to keep us afloat, and praying that my fears of his worsening drinking and potentially losing the Canterbury Park job would not come to fruition.

My fears were founded and less than three months after starting, he was fired. I never got the whole story from Erik as to what happened, but I know the truth in my heart. He was drinking too much. He would present his outlandish and grand ideas to his bosses. I know how pushy and belligerent he can be when he is drinking, and my best guess is that he bullied his way right out of his dream job. It was devastating and frustrating. I was overwhelmed with fear and indecision. But, I never drank. In fact, I continued to be repulsed by his drinking. Don't get me wrong, trying to bake banana bread and finding a bottle of liquor in the cupboard where the pans are kept threw me for a loop, and finding empty vodka bottles in various places, under the seat in his car, in his closet, in his sock drawer—that always was a challenge. But, instead of picking up the bottle to drink it, I dumped them out and called my sponsor. No one knew exactly what to do. People outside of the situation were often quick to tell me to just be done with him, but I did not know how to do that and keep Sawyer safe. It was during this time that my sponsor recommended Al-Anon.

♫Chapter Twenty♫

AL-ANON

What? Al-anon? For me? But I was a drunk! They are going to hate me there! She encouraged me and even attended my first meeting with me. Talk about feeling like a black sheep. Listening to all of their concerns and fears and frustrations, knowing I had put my loved ones through those very things and now facing it on the other side of the coin. I was what they called a "double winner," both loving an addict and being one. I did not feel like a winner. I felt spent. I felt trapped. I felt resentment, anger, sadness, fear. I also felt that I, as an alcoholic myself, needed to be compassionate and helpful to Erik and not abandon him. He constantly reminded me that if the roles were reversed, he would support me. So I felt guilty, too.

Surprisingly to me, Al-Anon has their own big blue book with the same Twelve Steps tweaked just a little bit. The whole program is the same. It is about focusing on yourself and your health and sanity, setting and enforcing healthy boundaries, and detaching with love. The comparison to being on an airplane when the oxygen masks come down and the order to put your own on first before other passengers was brought up. A person is simply incapable of truly caring for anyone else if their own house/life is not in order. I had to work on me. What? But HE is the problem. How is me working on myself going to stop this rollercoaster and get him sober? Well, it wasn't. Only he could get himself sober. But I could take care of myself and the kids, and get off that damn rollercoaster if I wanted to.

I can't recommend Al-Anon and its Steps and principles highly enough. If you love someone who is an addict or an alcoholic, GO. At least try a few meetings. At the very least, you will realize you are not alone. If you find a meeting that is just a bitch session and you feel worse and more hopeless leaving than you did walking in, find another meeting. Trust me, they are out there. Find one where the discussions are mainly centered around living in the solution, not the problem. We all know what the problem is. What we don't know, is how to fix it. The bottom line is the loved ones CAN'T fix it. The alcoholic or addict has to fix him or herself. The sooner we come to that realization, the sooner we can move forward with a life that we want; with or without the addict. Some people find strength in Al-Anon to stay with their loved one. Some decide to leave. Some are classic enablers and stuck but trying to find a way out. Some are codependent and so addicted/focused on the addict that their own well-being has long since taken a back seat. I never felt pressure to do, or not do anything. Just support and stories about what others had been through and how they got to a solution that worked for them.

I was really strapped for time, working three jobs and caring for the kids and the household as well as working my program. So, I did not become a regular Al-Anon attendee. I did, however, read that Al-Anon big book from cover to cover three times. It started making sense. My same character defects of fear, dishonesty, and people pleasing had come back front and center—insidiously. I was not drinking, but those same flaws were still causing me problems. Drinking was ruining my life—STILL. My sponsor and I worked the Twelve Steps, in Al-Anon style, focusing heavily on Steps Four through Seven, reviewing my defects and working on trying to release them. I was letting fear run my life, again. If I didn't get a handle on all of this and soon, a relapse was certain to happen. I was near my breaking point. Something had to give.

ᑕᔆᐯ Chapter Twenty-One ᕷᕲᑐ

DIVORCE #2

It sort of happened for me. Nick and Evelyn were with us for part of their summer break. As typical, Erik's drinking worsened while they were here. Add to that, he had been fired and had all the free time in the world. Instead of using that time to really enjoy his kids, he drank, and isolated, and spent so much time drinking and sleeping in the bedroom, alone. I tried to entertain the kids. Taking them to a theme park one day, the movies another, and I took Evelyn up to my sister's lake cabin with my other kids for several days.

That trip was a point of contention between Erik and me, because he and Nick were not invited due to their drinking and smoking pot, as well as some posts Nick had made on social media that had frightened my sister. They were no longer welcome until they got sober. Erik was furious and told me that, as his wife, and Nick's stepmother, I should tell my sister that either she invited all of us, or none of us. I felt and told him that this was unfair. She had a right to invite, or not, anyone she pleased. I had worked far too hard to restore my relationship with my sister and her family to let him ruin it for me. So, unlike the typical me, I did fight him on this. Calling my sister to tell her what was up, she recommended we just postpone the visit until Nick and Ev had gone back to Pennsylvania. But Evelyn really wanted to go and see the cousins whom she had come to adore. Nick understood the situation and was totally cool with us going without him and Erik, but Erik was angry. I decided to take the kids and go, anyway. Erik told me he did not think our relationship could sustain this. I took my chances, and secretly hoped he would just be gone when we came home. My father came to my sister's that week. It was unusual for him to take a several day break from farm work. I later learned he was there just in case Erik and Nick decided to follow us up there and cause trouble.

Erik wasn't gone when we returned. But he was even more angry and drunk. He wanted apologies to him and Nick from me. He wanted me to call my sister and tell her that her boundaries were unacceptable to me. He was trying to isolate me. I wasn't having it. The day before the kids were set to fly home, I was ready to go to my regular weekly health care provider recovery meeting. Erik threw a fit. He told me that if it was Tate and Olivia going away for a few months, I would never go to a meeting, I would skip it. He told me I was a terrible stepmother and had never loved Nick and Evelyn. His kids caught wind of this and fought for me. They defended me and assured me that I was not a horrible stepmother and that they loved me. Evelyn was hysterical and sobbing, telling me the only reason she ever came here was because of me and the other kids, not because of her dad. She screamed that he was a horrible person who had done her mother so wrong. Nick was determined to physically fight his Dad, he was angry at him for the present situation, but also due to his childhood abandonment issues and feelings that Erik always talked down to him and told him what to do and didn't listen and basically bullied him. Erik had been telling Nick to stop drinking, but he had no leg to stand on because he was drunk all the time. To Nick, all of Erik's words were hypocritical. I took Sawyer and wanted to take Evelyn to get out of the house, but she refused. She and Nick told me to just get out of there before it got worse. I packed a small overnight bag for Sawyer and myself as I had no idea what was in store next. I left to go to the meeting.

I did not actually go to the meeting, obviously. I was too nervous about what was going on at home between Erik and his son, with poor Evelyn right there. I spoke to their mother back in Pennsylvania. She asked me to call the police, which I did. I parked just two blocks away and texted with Evelyn constantly. She hid upstairs in one of the bedrooms while Nick and Erik had it out. The police came and apparently defused the situation. Erik's ex-wife called me back and told me it would be awesome—her word—if I could somehow get the kids out of there for the night to stay at an airport hotel so I could get them safely on the plane home early the next morning as planned.

Letting Evelyn know the plan, she and Nick hurriedly threw their belongings in their suitcases. I promised I would ship out any forgotten items. I parked around the corner, they ran to my car and we were off. Erik was stumbling about in the yard trying to come after us, yelling, confused. My son Tate, thankfully, was at camp that week. My daughter was over at a friend's house. I had packed a few things for her, as well. We picked her up and the five of us found a suite at a hotel by the airport and settled in. Everyone was so upset. Olivia was confused and trying to piece together what in the world had happened. Nick and Evelyn were both so angry at their dad. My adrenaline had kept me going for the day, but finally we all crashed. At four AM the next morning, I dropped Nick and Ev at the airport, hugging them so tightly through tears, wondering if this would be the last time I ever got to see those beautiful kids. I returned to the hotel where Olivia was sleeping with Sawyer, slept for a couple hours, and then took Sawyer to daycare and took Olivia with me to work. Yep—still had to work.

At the end of that workday, which was a Friday, we cautiously returned home. Erik was there, and he was angry. I typically avoid any confrontation and screaming matches, and tried to defuse the situation, but I was done. I screamed back. I yelled and cried and told him what his drinking had done to me, to the kids, to the family. I told him I felt betrayed and abandoned and that he had left me mentally long ago. I was hysterical, and Olivia had never heard me like that before. She slinked out of the house and called her dad, my ex-husband, who arranged for her to get dropped at his house to be away from the situation. But Sawyer was there, poor little Sawyer. I had a wedding reception planned the next day, and packed while Erik followed me around. I packed a lot—I knew I would never be coming back to the house as long as Erik was there. He did not catch wind of the excessive packing but continued to attempt to berate me about the situation the day before, about my sister, about everything bad in his life that he wanted to blame anyone else for. I was just in the line of fire. As we were leaving, he asked "why do you have to bring Sawyer?" Then he asked "are you ever coming home?" I didn't respond to either question. He then threatened suicide if we left.

We left.

As soon as we were on the road, I called Erik's old sponsor and Sawyer's Godfather Bob. I sobbed, pulled over, told him the situation, told him I was really worried about Erik but that I had to remove myself from the situation. Bob was in Chicago for the weekend. He asked some of his friends in the program if anyone could go do a welfare check, but since none of them knew Erik, they were afraid that he would not let them in or be receptive. So, Bob called the police for a welfare check. My husband, who had been sobbing and threatening suicide when I left, was found to be sitting on the couch drinking beer watching golf. That's the manipulation of alcoholics. Bob talked to Erik a couple of times over the phone, sent the police there one more time. I can only imagine what the neighbors thought, the police at our home three times in as many days.

Arriving up north for the wedding reception, my amazing parents once again were there to swoop in and save the day. They had pulled their fifth wheel camper up there as hotel rooms were scarce. We attended the lovely reception. Sawyer thought the camper was awesome. Everything was just his size! He and I slept on the pullout couch in the living area, Mom and Dad in the back bedroom. We spent a couple nights there in a campground, cooking, watching fun old comedies, and formulating a plan.

I contacted a divorce attorney. My sister graciously agreed to front the retainer. The attorney was a good one who charged a lot, had twenty-plus years' experience, and had a reputation for getting good outcomes for his clients during contentious divorces. I was expecting a fight, and I was putting on my armor. The biggest concerns for me were Sawyer, of course, and the house. I had bought that house in my name, had used my parents' money for the down payment, and had put my blood sweat and tears into making the house payments. Because of our financial situation, my credit had dropped from 830 to 514 at its worst. A second car had been repossessed and I paid out the nose to get it back. I had defaulted on a credit card and my wages had been garnished for six months until the 12K debt was paid. I had been working for a year to try to improve my credit, and it had risen 100 points but at 615, I would still be in no position to buy, or even rent, something reasonable. The house was important to me and to all three of my children.

I was scheduled to return to work in a few days, so I needed to get back to the area. My parents found a campground close to my home, and we caravanned there. We continued to enjoy our time, stressful as the situation was. Showering in shower houses, and cramped in the camper, the four of us managed to have some really good times. My sponsor was in Mexico during this time, but as always, was available via email. I contacted her and asked her if the kids and I could use her guest cottage for a while. She had offered it in the past when I was struggling with the situation with Erik, but I had yet to take her up on it. She responded right away that we could use it as long as needed. I picked up Olivia, Tate was still at camp, and Olivia, Sawyer, and I moved into a sweet little guest cottage on a small lake. I bought a pair of dress shoes and a work outfit at Target, as well as some diapers and wipes and a few items of clothing for Sawyer. Groceries, toilet paper, laundry soap were needed, so I bought small boxes and bottles of necessities. My parents maintained their campground spot and were close by. My mother stopped by the house where Erik was because I had left my nametag and stethoscope there. I was not about to go to the house and run into Erik. She told me he was very sad, apologizing, asking about me, asking her to tell me he loved me, but he was still drinking.

I was in contact with Bob, Erik's sponsor, daily. He was, again, a Godsend. He was working with Erik, going to the house daily, bringing him food and Gatorade and was working on getting him into treatment. Texts including insurance information, payment questions, issues about what to do with our three cats and dog if and when Erik went to treatment. After several days, Hazelden had an opening, and Bob took him there. I assured him that he didn't need to worry about the pets, because as soon as I knew Erik was admitted, the kids and I would be returning to our home.

What a relief! This time was different, though, because I had made up my mind. My allowing him back in the home was not going to happen. I was going to file for divorce. I had to, to save myself, my children, my finances. If by chance it also worked to serve as his rock bottom and saved his life that was just an added bonus. I was not counting on that, however. I had learned enough in Al-Anon and lived that life for long enough that it was clear that "nothing changes if nothing changes."

I served him divorce papers while he was in treatment, within the first week. This was done after careful consideration and discussion with his counselor. We agreed it would be best and safest if he got the news there, where he was surrounded by support. It was not an easy decision, because I still loved him very much and still wanted him to get better and still really missed and longed for the Erik I had first known.

Back at home, we settled into a routine and peaceful existence. I opened a separate bank account for all of my direct deposits. I finally knew where my money was going and began to get a handle on the finances. My credit continued to improve, though slowly. I was able to work and return home knowing that it would be my sanctuary, there would be no booze, no belligerent husband or sobbing emotional wreck of a husband. It was just me and the kids. Everyone was incredibly relieved.

Erik attempted to contact me, but I did not respond. I went up to Hazelden only once to meet him and his counselor, and the meeting went horribly, in my opinion. He went between sad and attempting to manipulate and control me, and had to be redirected by his counselor several times. He begged me not to give up on him. I assured him I hadn't given up; but that I would no longer be financially responsible for him and that he had to learn to stand on his own two feet.

Five months, to the date, from signing the divorce papers, our divorce was final. I was awarded sole custody and the house and my tiny retirement fund. I agreed to continue to pay his health insurance for a few months, cover half of his car payment and all of the car insurance. No spousal maintenance or child support was awarded to either of us. He was required to begin using Soberlink, a device that is quite convenient, works with his phone, and he does a photo breathalyzer three times daily, with results sent to me. He was awarded a few hours of visitation with Sawyer weekly, provided he stayed sober. Erik did not put up much of a fight, legally.

He has maintained his sobriety thus far, but as I write this we are only several weeks out from finalization of the divorce. I have made sure he sees Sawyer much more frequently than the court order states, because as long as he is sober, he and Sawyer are good for each other. Every kid deserves to have a father present if possible, but a sober and safe father. Erik is that today.

Utilizing accountability tools, such as an ignition interolock and/or Soberlink has proven to be invaluable to me, both as an alcoholic, and now as the loved one of an alcoholic. If you are trying to claw your way back out of the depths and attempting to earn back trust, I have found these products priceless. I receive instant email results regarding Erik's breath tests. In our divorce paperwork, it is clear that if he relapses, his time with Sawyer ends. In my own situation several years ago, the ignition interlock and random observed urine tests provided security and proof to my children, to my ex-husband, and to my medical licensing board that I was sober. The services take away some of the fear, the constant wondering if the alcoholic is drinking. If clear boundaries and consequences for a violation are set, the additional accountability can provide a significant deterrence. Active alcoholics, by nature, are liars. Often, by the time one truly embraces sobriety, nobody believes a word that comes out of their mouths. With these tools, an alcoholic in recovery can actually *prove* they are sober, rather than just saying it and expecting people to believe it.

I still love Erik dearly. I am very proud of him for staying sober so far. I will catch myself laughing and enjoying conversations with him more and more. The old Erik is back, and even better. He is working his program, seeing his sponsor, going to meetings, has even begun to sponsor others, and has done the jail orientation to begin bringing meetings there. He is spending quality time with Sawyer, and with me. He has taken a job managing the childcare at a YMCA and seems to enjoy it. He talks of going back to school for a teaching degree. He slips up and attempts to control me sometimes; he has asked me if I would cover his child support for Nick and Ev for a few months, which I refused. He also asked if I would help him financially if he goes back to school, which I also refused. Erik has never managed money, and I believe he truly needs to provide for himself, on his own, without using me or anyone else to bail him out. I slip up sometimes and tell him what I think he wants to hear or avoid saying things to try to prevent hurting his feelings. But we have been able to have some meaningful discussions about our defects and our attempts to better ourselves. It is very nice to have him back on the recovery train.

Tate and Olivia, at present, have no interest in seeing him. He does not come to pick up Sawyer or see him when the kids are here. My parents, particularly my father, have made clear that they also have no desire to see him. My mother, like me, has a very tender heart and she is hopeful, for the kids' sake that he will stay sober and find happiness. It will take a long time to gain trust back. I know that it took a couple of years for my children to fully trust me after I got sober. Maybe they will begin to trust him as the months add up (IF they add up) with Erik staying sober, maybe they will not. My kids are my first priority, and I will do nothing that threatens their happiness. They have gone through too much already in their young lives.

I can't predict the future, and my program teaches me to take things one day at a time, which I do. Erik may relapse; his history is suggestive of that. But maybe he won't. Maybe he will become a teacher; maybe not. Maybe he will stay sober and be able to be present in the lives of his children, perhaps not. Maybe, down the road a year or two, if he stays sober, we can try again. I have a glimmer of hope that we could once again be a great team someday and raise our son together. But for now, things are peaceful and stable and I will not give that up for anything. I have no interest in dating anyone else right now, as my experiences with men have been less than ideal. I also need to stand on my own two feet for a while, and reconnect with myself. It feels good.

ᶜᵉᴼ Chapter Twenty-Two ᵉᴼᵕ

FROM TATE

I am my mother's oldest child, almost seventeen at this point. I guess drinking was a problem for many years. I do remember some fights between my parents before their divorce. There was a lot of yelling, throwing things, I tried to get in the middle of it a couple of times to stop it but it didn't change anything so I stopped trying.

When I was about ten, I remember a trip to Florida with my mom and sister to meet our grandparents, aunt and uncle, and cousins there for Christmas. Although I did not know that Mom's drinking was the cause, the trip included several weird situations.

The first was that on the way to the airport, Mom didn't seem to know how to get there. I remember she drove in one particular loop three times. Mom had me call Grandma to help us get there. Later I found out that Grandma was really concerned because she knew there was clearly a problem if Mom didn't know where the *airport was, which she had been to many times. At that time, I didn't really know what was going on, and I wasn't scared, it just seemed strange.*

I think it was the second night of our trip, I remember that Mom took us into the small bathroom when Aunt Crystal was trying to break into the room. Mom told us that Crystal was trying to take us away. We hid in there for what seemed like a couple of hours, it felt like a really long time but it was probably only about fifteen minutes until Crystal stopped banging on the door.

I believe the very next day, it was confusing, because Mom told us we were getting packed up to go somewhere else in Florida. I felt OK with it, because I thought Crystal was bad at that point and that Mom was right. Before we could leave, Crystal, Paul, and my Great Aunt Carol came to our hotel. I remember my Mom's Aunt Carol talking to my Mom, who was in her bed by that time. Carol was crying, she didn't want Mom to leave and take us. Carol told Mom she didn't want us to get in an accident and I was really confused about this because my mom had driven us around our whole life. I didn't understand what drinking really meant. After that day, I only saw my Mom two or three times the rest of the trip, Mom was in bed, and we swam and went to Disneyworld with our cousins and had a great time.

I can't remember why we were driving home one day, I think it was the end of a school day and Mom had picked us up. We were about to turn off the highway into our neighborhood, and Mom took a left turn at a bad time and another car was coming and almost hit us. That is when I started to become really scared riding with Mom in the car.

At one point, Mom had been in bed for three straight days. I knew there was a problem, but I didn't know what the problem was. I talked to my sister Olivia about it; I knew there was something seriously wrong. Mom never came to eat. I made some noodles for Mom during that time, but she wouldn't eat them. My feelings were hurt, I was pretty sad. I wanted her to eat. I wanted her to be OK. My sister and I made ourselves our own snacks. The huge size of our house made everything worse. It was lonely. Mom even called us in sick to school a few times and sometimes she would lie to us and tell us that there was no school that day.

Olivia and I hid in my walk in closet and called Grandma and Grandpa. I told them that Mom had been in bed for three days, wasn't cooking, wasn't eating, wasn't talking much and always sounded really tired and drowsy when she would talk. So, they got in their car and came. I was very happy that they decided to come. It wasn't lonely in the house anymore. They cooked, they took us to school, basically did everything a parent would do, and I was very relieved. Then Mom went to detox.

After detox, she came home but still drank. Grandma and Grandpa kept staying with us. I got good at trying to find her hidden bottles and would sometimes spy on Mom to try to find them. If I found one, I gave it to Grandma and Grandpa.

She went to treatment, Grandma and Grandpa stayed with us. We went to visit Mom at treatment. I enjoyed how peaceful it was both at home and at treatment, but I was never hopeful that she would change.

Mom dropped us off at our therapist, Jonathan's office. I was really scared on the drive there, Mom was swerving around and she ran over a curb on the way and in the parking lot and almost hit the car parked next to us. I knew she had a bag in the front seat with bottles in it. Mom sent us in to therapy alone. She stayed in the car. I wanted her to come in, I yelled at her to come in with us, but she wouldn't. I got mad and slammed the door and Olivia and I went in. Then I told Jonathan that Mom was drunk. I asked him if he could come to the car with us. He said he would.

We all went out to the car; I opened the passenger's door, and grabbed the bottles out of Mom's hands and gave them to Jonathan. Jonathan said that we couldn't leave with Mom. He called my dad who came to pick us up. I was so angry through the whole thing. I was happy to see Dad, though. I told my Dad everything that had been going on. I had been angry at Dad in the past, and had been on Mom's side. Now, I was firmly on Dad's side.

At that point, we moved in with Dad and his pregnant girlfriend, Tiffany. We had to switch schools, which was OK. At first, things were really good at Dad's. As time passed, they began to drink more and fight a lot.

Before Mom went to her last rehab, she had a couple of boyfriends. The first was Michael. Nobody liked Michael. I didn't like Michael. He was a cheater. He was just a bad person in general. When Mom broke up with Michael, I was very happy. He does not deserve any more words than this.

Then came Mark. He was a person Mom decided to date right after they both left treatment. He was a good person, except when he was on cocaine. Mom had already started drinking again, and Mark did things with us, like taking me to baseball practice. All four of us did things together, too. That relationship ended badly.

Mom's last treatment was in Florida, and it was long. She was gone for three months. We lived with Dad during that time. I didn't think Mom would ever change. I didn't really even want to see her when she came back. It always made me feel better that she had a parenting supervisor and the Intoxalock.

It took me a very long time to trust Mom, probably a couple of years. The main way that I gained trust back was with time. Mom was doing what she was supposed to be doing with meetings and just not drinking. I am really proud of her and what she has done these past few years, and my confidence that she won't drink again is very high. I don't even worry about it or think about it much anymore.

Unfortunately, I can't really say the same about Dad right now. He is an alcoholic, too. He took a trip to rehab about a year ago now after his second DWI. He has been sober about a year, and he seems to have found more happiness than he had before. I think that's the way you can stay sober. He seems to have found happiness by surrounding himself with other people. I have learned how important happiness and finding other things to fill your time is when you give up drinking.

After watching all of this, drinking is something I plan to avoid. I am going to be aware that I have a personality where I get attached to things very easily, and I have to be aware of that. I guess that means I have an addictive personality, and I come by it naturally. Alcohol can ruin every aspect of a persons' life from relationships to jobs to money to your house, it can literally affect every part of your life. Mom lost her house, her job, her relationship with her family and with her kids. She got it back, but it took a lot of time and hard work. She had to give up what she had been using for pleasure and happiness for twenty years and she says it's the hardest thing she ever has done, and I believe it. My dad lost his job, his girlfriend, and my trust. I don't fully trust him yet. My ex stepfather has truly lost everything due to his drinking and the decisions he made due to drinking. He has lost his relationship with his kids, his wife, and his lifestyle that Mom was paying for. I don't want to ever fight that battle, so if I don't start the battle, I won't ever have to fight it.

Chapter Twenty-Three

FROM OLIVIA

I've always loved my mom, from the start to the end. Even during the times where she was so lost within her drinking habits. Even during the times where I'd have to sit next to her in bed so she could feel a little less lonesome. I knew she feared that she would lose me along with the love I have for her, but I did everything in my power to make sure she could have at least a little hope.

There have been many, many times throughout my life when I told myself that my mom was never going cut off her drinking habits. I love my mom with all my heart, but I still knew that my faith in her sobriety was slowly decaying.

One of the toughest things that I had to go through almost every day was how often I was lied to. I knew many places where my mom would hide away her big bottles of either wine or vodka. In her closet behind clothes, in her drawers, in a large basket where we put our blankets, under her bed—the list goes on.

*I've looked my mom in the eyes and I have asked,
"Mom, are you drinking again? I found this bottle in one of
your hiding spots." She'd look me in the eyes and tell me,
"No Olivia, I'm not drinking. This bottle you found is old."*

*Usually after I was told that the bottle was old, I'd
feel relieved. I was only seven- years-old or so, I wasn't
ever able to feel skeptical about much. Not until my mom's
transitions to rehab and relapse became a pattern.*

*Later on I was finally able to recognize that what
was going on with my mom wasn't what some would
consider "Normal." For a while I was too young to let it
affect me, not until I was able to look back at what has
happened in my life and have been able to recognize that
my mom needed help.*

*During that time, my faith was decaying in both of
my parents. Both of them were addicts, fighting back and
forth while throwing Tate and me in the middle of each
argument. I was still too young to know that alcohol could
potentially kill my parents, but I knew that it hurt them.*

*For a while Tate and I had to live through having to
choose sides between parents. They'd fight so much that it
created an atmosphere where we had to choose to either
support mom or support dad. I'd always ask myself, "Do I
choose to be on my mom's side with my dad being upset, or
do I choose to be on my dad's side and have my mom feel
even more alone?" I never could even choose between my
parents. Both Tate and I decided that we wouldn't pick any
side.*

Times like these are sometimes painful to remember. Both of the people I most looked up to were fighting and angry. In the process, my mom dated other guys and my dad dated other girls. All of it was a mess.

I never knew what I was supposed to do. Often times I'd believe the situation with my parents was my fault. I had no idea how to change what was happening. So I started to hide from everything. I'd stay in my room a lot and if I heard fighting I'd find someplace to hide. When I hid, I'd usually draw to distract myself. My grandmother named me the "invisible child" once people noticed how often I'd disappear. That was my only way to cope with the toxic environment I lived in.

I was a prisoner in my own house. I lived in two different houses of course, but I'd always hide in both. I had to live through lots of fear. Alcoholism shaped all the downfalls throughout my childhood. I didn't know what or who to blame, my parents, the alcohol, or even myself. I was too young to know who was to blame.

I am still lucky because during that time I still had the support of my grandparents, my aunts and uncles, my cousins, and my brother. But everyone but Tate lived far away. I mainly had the support of my brother, only because I never had much of a way to talk to those other family members.

Tate was brave. He protected me so much during those few years. If he hadn't been around, I would have no idea about what my life would be like now. I'm just glad I don't have to find out.

Aside from this, I'm very proud of my mom. Trust may take years to build, but only seconds to break. I'm so glad my mom is over five years sober. A lot of my faith has built back up again as well. Now my life is so much different, I have the best mom ever.

She was one of the only people who was truly there for me when I went through seventh grade, when I got diagnosed with severe depression and anxiety. New downfalls happened that year. But my mom is the biggest reason I made it through.

In conclusion, there have been times where I thought my mom would never get better. But, she not only made it past her alcohol addiction, she also became ten times stronger. I'm so happy for her and I'm so glad to have such an amazing and supportive mom.

Chapter Twenty-Four

FROM MOM

K*arla, where do I start?*
It has been painful for the whole family.
First of all, the learning curve on Alcoholism was immense.
I thought my love and faith in Karla was the right way to
be. My husband and her sister were angry and did not
share my tender heart feelings. I am a fantastic enabler and
at the same time the one who probably taught her the most
about being a people pleaser. So, I had a lot to learn.

Fear—the call from her sister that Karla was in
SERIOUS trouble with her drinking really caused fear.
What was happening? How could I help? What should I
do? (I'm a nurse, and Nurses fix things.) So, we hopped in
the car (several different times) and made the four hour
drive to her house not knowing what we would find. And
then there were her two beautiful children. Someone had to
be there for them. Because she and their Dad (who is also
an alcoholic) were in the process of divorcing, we weren't
always sure what to do or where to be.

Sadness—I think I felt overwhelmed with sadness when we found her in an almost comatose, emaciated state. All she would or could consume was continual sips of brandy. She wanted me to let her die, actually, begged me to let her die.

Action—the nurse in me said, "not on my watch!" So, off to detox we went, then on to Hazelden. We stayed with her children (a blessing for us, as it was something constructive to do.) And I attended the family session. I figured the angry members of the family needed this much more than I did, but I was wrong. I learned so much! I did go through her house and threw out all the hidden alcohol I found. She had some fantastic hiding places!

Family strife—my husband and I fought (verbally). This is not the way we are. We were dividing the family. And I was stubborn, I wouldn't back down.

First recovery meeting—I attended it with Karla. One of the other members of the group took me aside and informed me that it was nice that I supported her at her first meeting, but from here on out, it was "none of my business." He was right. I learned I did not cause, could not control, or could not cure her alcoholism. This was her ballgame. I could love her, but it had to be unconditional love. "No more drinking" was not related to my love. And I could not bail her out of whatever she got into due to her drinking. She had to deal. I had to go home.

Relapse—Ughhh. This time we received a call from the children's therapist, stating they had initiated an intervention for Karla. This time, her children's Dad was involved and helped care for the children. Into detox and rehab, again. Out of fear for the children's safety, I had talked with them about not getting into the car with their mother if she was drinking. They told the therapist that she was in the parking lot, drinking while they were in session with him. Thus, the intervention took place.

On February 12, 2012, my niece ended her life. This was so devastating for all of us, and it really added to my fears for Karla. We could see her spiraling down as she grieved for her cousin. My niece was very close to Karla when they were growing up, and it was a frightful experience. Once again, fear!

My feelings—there were so many other incidents that I could include, but the point is, it didn't just happen and get fixed in a day. I felt physically ill with worry much of the time for a couple years. My feelings were all mixed up. I'm not a cryer, but I felt on the verge of tears most of the time. This was my first born, my beautiful talented, smart daughter, the apple of my eye. What had I done to her that drove her to this state? What I learned, I found very hard to put into practice. I read a lot. It was kind of my escape. And I worried whether I was physically up to raising her children if necessary. I was afraid. And I didn't (couldn't) sleep. So, many nights I just prayed. There was nothing else I could think of to do.

Karla is five years sober now. But it is still on my mind frequently. If I don't hear her voice for over a week, then I wonder if she is OK. I'm sleeping better, so, I guess I have learned to let go a bit. But, it's a continual challenge for me. Life is so precious, but it can hurt so much. So, I pray and I reach out to anyone else struggling with addiction. Maybe they will feel hopeful when our story is shared. It's not easy, but it's worth it!

ᏣᎠChapter Twenty-FiveᐁᏯ

FROM DAD

I can't imagine what life would be like if we had lost Karla. It was very real and very close to happening. For her growing up years, except for the first ten months (when she was a colicky, fussy baby), she was a parent's dream. She was an early achiever and always seemed to do her best. Friends would comment about how proud we must be of her (which we were) and that we must really push her hard. I don't think we pushed her hard but we did try to reward her after a job well done. (Maybe that was more pushing than we intended). She did very well in Elementary and High school and graduated from college in three years. Then on to PA school. Friends said to us, "now, you're done." The same was said when she married. Our stock answer was we don't know if you're ever done. I'm glad that's the way we answered, because we were not done.

I'm sure we missed some signs with Karla growing up that could have been a warning to us, like having trouble sleeping and the ability to handle her liquor so well *for a young person (5'6" 130# and twenty-one). She could easily last longer in a bar and I'm 6 ft and 185# and was about forty-five-years-old at that time.*

I remember her saying once; she wondered why the boys didn't seem to want her. That made me feel bad, but I remember when i was in school some of the girls in my class were so far more successful and involved in activities that I was intimidated. I felt I would have been turned down anyway and maybe that's how they felt.

So, in saying this, I think Karla may have settled for not only one husband that wasn't good for her but after rehab, another one that was even worse. I'm so relieved that she is now divorced. Her second husband was going to bankrupt her and put her back on booze.

There is a certain amount of good which has come out of this bad situation and that is we have three super grand kids which we have been able to be with a lot. I hope they will feel the same as the years go by.

I find myself bragging more about Karla now than I ever did in the past due to her own decisions to change her life. I can also see how important her support group is to her and how she supports others. I feel they are able to do more for each other than we as parents can.

❧Chapter Twenty-Six❧

FROM MY SISTER

Who are you? Who is the shell of a person that used to be my sister, who used to be my best friend? Your eyes are so dark and so hollow, your words are so hateful and mean. You lie—all of the time. I want to help and love you, but you can't be helped. You have to help yourself. But you won't. Your disease which causes you to hate, lie, and cheat has made it impossible for me to continue being near you. So I quit you. I quit answering your calls, I quit hoping you'd get healthy, I quit caring about you, I quit acknowledging I even had a sister. The only thing I cared about was making sure your children were okay, but I didn't care if I ever saw your face again, because seeing you hurt. And knowing you were slowly killing yourself was killing me. I didn't want to care and I didn't want it to hurt the day someone called me and told me you had died. So I quit you. And it was easier and better that way.

Life continued to go on. Without you. Almost as if you had died.

Until one day, you came back! Clean. Sober. Clear. Genuine. I was able to meet you. The new you. The real you. For the first time, ever. And I liked you. So we started to get to know each other, as new friends do, and in time, you became a trusted friend to me and you became my sister again. And it's really scary. Just writing this, my heart feels so much pressure; my stomach is in knots, because of the awful memories. Because there's always something in the back of my mind telling me that I could lose you again to this disease. And it haunts my dreams, and it makes me cry. But as long as I don't dwell on those feelings and nightmares and push myself to live for what IS today, I am blessed to have my sister back and will love you for what IS today and pray for a good tomorrow.

Peace and Serenity

"God, Grant Me the Serenity to Accept the Things I Cannot Change, the Courage to Change the Things I Can, and the Wisdom to Know the Difference"

ᒃ᠊ᢀChapter Twenty-Seven᠋ᢀᢀ

WHAT NOW?

Do you hear it? The fear? It is in the words of those I love the most. It is in my own words. This alcoholism—it is always going to be with me. I get but a daily reprieve from its ravages. I am not cured. I can't predict the future with certainty. I can't say without a doubt I will never drink again. But I can say that, today, I will not drink. Today, I will work my program. Today, I will ask for help from God and my sober support network, and I will be available for those in need. Today, I will nurture those relationships dear to me because I never want to put anyone through the horrors of alcoholism again. I never want to *experience* those horrors again. If each day, I live by being genuine and present, and each day I can commit to not drinking, then God willing, those "one day at a time's will continue.

Do you also hear the guilt? My words, the words of my loved ones, everyone seems to have terrible guilt about what they did, should have done, didn't do, somehow trying to figure out who or what was to blame for my alcoholism. The truth is it was nobody's fault but mine. I chose to take that first drink when I was young. But something in me, a defect, or physiologic response, led to an addiction at which point I could not simply stop and at that point, it wasn't even my fault anymore. I didn't grow up wanting to be an alcoholic. No one chooses to be an addict. There is still a huge stigma about alcoholism. Is it a disease? An allergy? A moral failing? Nobody, including me, knew what to do. And the most horrid part is that this is an illness of denial. I am not aware of another affliction in life that tries to convince those who have it that they don't!

I wrote this book in an attempt to reveal what is going on inside the brain of an active alcoholic. But more importantly that no matter how much has been lost or destroyed, there is still hope as long as you have your life. I truly believe that if I can become sober and live a happy and fulfilled life without alcohol, *anyone can*. There are millions upon millions of people out there with stories like mine. Many, without happy endings as alcoholism and addiction continue to claim lives every day. Yes, my life has been filled with mistakes and I have hurt a lot of people. I have wasted precious time and was not the mother my children deserved. But with time, commitment, and the help of God and many people, I have turned it around into something wonderful and better than I could have ever imagined. You can, too. Or your loved ones can. Or your coworker in the next cubicle can. Recovery is possible!

Since completion of this book, my ex-husband Jim has celebrated a year of recovery. I presented him his one-year chip and it was probably the coolest experience the two of us have had in years. Both sober, we have been able to effectively parent our children in a collaborative, caring, and loving manner. I want the best for him, and I believe he wants that for me as well. We are actually friends now. I have invited him to join my weekly healthcare recovery meeting, which he says has been very helpful to his recovery. We sat down and read this book together, as I wanted him to be comfortable with all that I was "putting out there." We have realized that we had a really good thing – a good marriage, the world on a string. Alcohol destroyed it. We *allowed* alcohol to poison us and destroy our marriage and lives in the process. We went from love to hate due to the drinking. Now, in sobriety, we are friends. We support each other and our efforts to stay sober, and to parent our children. I no longer look with fear at my phone if he calls. I actually answer and know that we will have a civil and pleasant conversation, even if the topic is a difficult one.

Erik has now celebrated 9 months of sobriety. This is the longest he can recall being sober in his adult life. He is back to the kind and supportive man I once knew. He is working a solid program of recovery. He continues to work at the YMCA in childcare, and is actively pursuing a job with the US Postal service. He is learning how to manage his own finances for the first time in his life. He has had to lose a great deal and learn what it is like to feel stress and pressure regarding money and employment prospects. He seems to have grasped the enormity of the financial strain that was put on me during our marriage. He is very active in Sawyer's life. He has restored his relationship with his son, Nick, and continues to try to be patient with Evelyn who is still not ready for him. He has stepped up and is responsible for getting Sawyer off the bus from school and caring for him while I work urgent care shifts. Now, when he takes care of Sawyer, he is present. They go to the park, they go to the store, they play. They don't just watch TV. Tate and Olivia have now begun to trust him and have some enjoyable times with him as well. It is a slow process, but he is once again my very best friend and I am so proud of him.

I can't predict the future for Jim, Erik, myself, or any other alcoholic or addict out there. But for today, all three of us are sober, and it is remarkable. Stunning, actually. And it is a beautiful thing.

It took nearly dying to really live. It took nearly losing everything to appreciate what I have. It took nearly destroying the relationships with those I loved to recreate them into something wonderful. I did not know what I had until it was gone. Now I am fully aware of the blessings, undeserved, that I have been granted in my life. The grace I have been shown by God, my loved ones, my recovery community and my work amazes me. There is a reason I am still here. My survival has to matter! Yet I am not out of the woods. Nobody in recovery is out of the woods. Ever.

As my dear friend Jeff says, "We are all on the same road in recovery—the same journey—going in the same direction but at different points on the road. Some several years down the road, some just a few hours or days. But we are all the same short distance from the ditch." My first and most important job every day is to not take that first drink. More important than being a mother, or daughter, or sister, or PA, or eating, or sleeping, or anything else. As long as I don't take that first drink, everything else is going to be manageable. There is nothing in this world, good or bad, that I couldn't make worse by drinking. And nothing in this world, good or bad, that I would make better by drinking.

I cannot afford to become complacent, because that's when this thing will swoop in. And destroy all that is dear to me. And kill me.

And I will be damned if I allow that.

Literally.

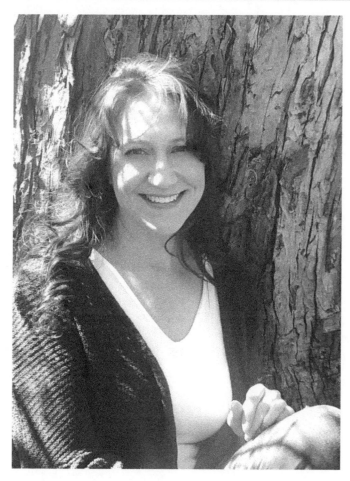

❦About the Author❧

K arla Juvonen is a Physician Assistant practicing in the state of Minnesota, where she lives with her three children, three cats, one dog, and one ex-husband. She enjoys reading, baking, playing the piano, and above all, spending time with her family. She previously enjoyed copious amounts of cheap liquor, which she has now replaced with Diet Coke by the liter. She is very active in her recovery community, leading meetings, working with other addicts and alcoholics, and speaking at treatment centers with regularity. She has learned how precious life is and has become incredibly grateful for second chances.

Sources/References

If you are a healthcare worker or provider, in recovery or with a desire to recover, and would like to anonymously communicate with other healthcare providers in recovery, please check out my website and blog at: www.hcprecovery.com.

To contact me directly, Karla Juvonen via email: Karla@hcprecovery.com.

The Big Book of Alcoholics Anonymous – 4th Edition. Copyright 2019 by Alcoholics Anonymous World Services.

Drop the Rock: Removing Character Defects – Steps 6-7. By Bill P., Todd W., and Sara S. Copyright 2005 by Hazelden Foundation.

Drop the Rock: The Ripple Effect – Using Step 10 to Work Steps 6 and 7 Every Day. By Fred H. Copyright 2016 by Hazelden Foundation.

The Four Agreements – A Practical Guide to Personal Freedom. By Don Miguel Ruiz. Copyright Amber-Allen Publishing.

Intoxalock – www.intoxalock.com

SmartStart – www.smartstartinc.com

Soberlink – www.soberlink.com

Suicide hotline – 1-800-273-8255

National Drug Hotline (addiction and alcoholism) – 1-888-633-3239.

AA website – www.aa.org

NA website – www.na.org

Al-Anon website – www.al-anon.org

Alateen website – www.al-anon.org